Contents

About the Author

Barry Groves lives with his wife, Monica, in a small village in the Cotswolds. Originally trained as an electronic engineer, he was commissioned in the Royal Air Force, with which he served until 1982.

In 1962 he developed a personal interest in the role of food types in the aetiology of obesity. When he retired from the RAF, at the age of forty-five, he took up full-time research, later broadening the scope of his studies to include the relationship between diet and other modern diseases such as heart disease and cancers.

He realised that the perceived wisdoms, both of low-calorie dieting for weight loss and 'healthy eating' for the control of heart disease, were seriously flawed. The public were being misled, largely, it seemed, to increase the profits of commercial interests.

He began to give talks and lectures, at first locally and then, increasingly, over an ever-wider area. However, he realised that to reach more people a book was needed. In 1988 he bought a computer, taught himself to use it, and began to write.

He is a columnist, writing about dietary and health matters for his local paper, *The Oxford Times*, and has written a column for the *Weekend Financial Times*. He has also been published in the *Lancet* in Britain and *The Townsend Letter for Doctors and Patients* in the USA.

He has served as a councillor on the West Oxfordshire District Council, where he was Chairman of the Environmental Health Committee. And with a long-term interest in energy conservation, he and his wife designed and built their own solar-heated house.

In 1982, he took up archery. With his compound bow, he became the British Clout Archery Champion in 1987. He retained this championship in the subsequent four years and in 1994, holding all the British records in this discipline from 1989 to 1992.

In 1992 he entered the British Flight Archery Championships, winning at his first attempt with a British record. He has successfully defended this championship every year since and taken a further ten British records. He has also won eleven International Gold Medals and seven World Records.

Introduction

One must attend in medical practice not primarily to plausible theories but to experience combined with reason.
HIPPOCRATES

The Eat Fat, Get Thin diet

What should you be eating to reduce to and maintain a normal weight? There are so many apparently conflicting theories about diet. *Eat Fat, Get Thin* looks at our evolution to see what foods we are adapted to eat. It discusses the reasons why we alone, as a species, get fat, and it explores the history of slimming over the past 130 years. It also contains yet another dietary regime. It may seem a revolutionary regime but it is not a new one. For more than a century it has been proven to be safe and effective, both in epidemiological studies and in clinical trials. It is a dietary regime that is both natural and healthy but more than that, as it does not restrict calorie intake, it is easy to maintain – and it works, simply because it is based on the natural diet for our species.

The origin of the Eat Fat, Get Thin diet

Eat Fat, Get Thin began in 1962 when I was working in Singapore with the Royal Air Force. We had a problem, my wife and I: we were overweight. We had tried all the usual ways to lose weight: cutting calories, eating inert fillers, taking appetite suppressants, wearing sweaty clothes, indeed we tried just about every weight-loss idea going, with results that were decidedly short term.

The first moment of revelation came, sudden and unexpected, when I was walking through the bustling Changi Market. I saw a second-hand bookstall and, being an inveterate browser, stopped to see what was on offer. One small paperback stood out. That book changed our lives – and our figures – for good. The book advocated what we thought was impossible: an *unrestricted*-calorie diet for weight loss. It said in so many words: eat as many calories as you like, and the pounds will fall away. Because this proposition seemed so out of keeping with all we had read up to that time, we decided to see what the diet could do for us. To our astonishment, it worked – and it has gone on working now for over thirty-seven years.

Then the questions began: If an unrestricted-calorie diet can achieve such results, why are all the books and magazine articles in favour of calorie-controlled diets? I began my research and the answers came. All the evidence I found persuaded me that low-calorie dieting is a snare for the overweight and a delusion for all concerned.

As I read on and on, it dawned on me that a vast 'health' industry made a very good living out of the business of offering expensive solutions for the problems, so they said, of keeping ourselves slim and fit. All those advertisements on television – eat this special food, try that diet – could they have anything to do with the profit motive?

Later we questioned whether the diet we were following, which was relatively high in animal fat, might be dangerous in terms of increased risk of heart disease. And so, when I retired from the Royal Air Force in 1982, I devoted myself full time to researching the healthiness of 'healthy eating'. All too soon I found that, contrary to what we read in newspapers and magazines, and hear on the radio and TV, there is very little evidence to show that 'healthy eating' is good for either the health or the figure.

The 10 September 1994 edition of the *British Medical Journal* published two papers about obesity. One expressed grave reservations about the effectiveness of present dietary treatments for obesity while the other asked: should we treat obesity?

Being overweight has affected a small proportion of the population for centuries but clinical obesity was relatively rare until this century. Indeed obesity remained at a fairly stable low level until about 1980. Then its incidence began to increase dramatically. By 1992 one in every ten people in Britain was obese; a mere five years later that figure had almost doubled. In the USA the situation is even worse: by 1991 one in three adults was overweight. That is an increase of eight per cent of the population over just one decade, despite the fact that, as a commentary in the 15 July 1994 edition of the *Lancet* pointed out, Americans spend a massive $33 billion a year on 'slimming', as well as taking more exercise, and eating fewer calories and less fat than they did ten years ago. There is now a pandemic of increasing weight across the industrialised world.

It may be hard to believe, but this has occurred in the face of increasing knowledge, awareness, and education about obesity, nutrition and exercise. It has happened despite the fact that calorie intake has gone down by twenty per cent over the past ten years and exercise clubs have mushroomed. More people are cutting calories now than ever before in their history, yet more of them are becoming overweight. Why should this be?

The fact is that obesity does not afflict any other animal species. Wherever you look around the world, you will not find an overweight animal in the wild. Animals in their natural habitat are either hunters or hunted. If they were overweight, either they would have difficulty catching their prey, or they would be easier for the carnivores to catch. Thus an overweight animal would not survive for long. It is true that there are animals which naturally carry a large amount of fat: whales, for example, who need it as insulation against the cold Arctic waters, and bears, who store fat as a food reserve for hibernation in the winter. But this is not obesity. Whether it is a herd of cows, a hive of bees, a pride of lions, or any other animal species, all the animals in a species are essentially the same size and none is obese.

Obesity is also noticeably absent in primitive human cultures. The only animals to get fat are 'civilised' man and his pets. And that is highly significant. The reason cannot be genetic or hereditary, as some argue. If it were, obesity would have plagued us for generations. And it cannot be simply that we eat too much, although many of us do. If an abundance of food were the cause, other animals with an ample food supply would also get fat, yet they don't. And if that were the reason, cutting calories would work; it doesn't, except in the short term.

Obesity is big business

Jules Hirsch, of Rockefeller University, New York, observed in the 1994 Herman Award Lecture to the American Society for Clinical Nutrition:

> The public must understand that all current methods, from thigh creams to stomach staples, are like gropes in the dark, and as such, are either totally ineffectual or are no more than counterforces to an incompletely understood regulatory disorder. There are no cures at this time.

In this he was wrong, as this book will show. However, Dr Hirsch put his finger on a major stumbling block when he said:

The ambiguities inherent in [the] problem . . . have led to the growth of a flourishing industry for weight control. The basic tenets of this industry are that there are commercially available programs that can safely lower body weight more easily than those of competitors and unlike their competitors, once the weight is lost, it will remain that way for ever. On this basis an endless set of new products, new diets and drug interventions play legal tag with governmental regulatory agencies while reaping profit from a public desperate for answers.

In this Hirsch was right: the many commercial interests that rely on overweight people to make a living compound today's weight epidemic. Walk into any large newsagent's shop and count the number of slimming magazines. Then add the number of slimming articles in women's magazines. Add also the slimming clubs and manufacturers of slimming products: foods, counselling, exercise equipment and clothes. 'Slimming' is an enormous money-spinner. You may not have realised it, but the first concern of the slimming businesses is not helping people to slim. They are like any other business, working to make a profit, to increase their market share and, above all, to stay in business. If they published a dietary regime which really did slim you as easily and permanently as they all claim, would you need to buy the next edition or pay the next club fee? No: doing so would be tantamount to committing commercial suicide.

Unreasonable regimes

Over the past twenty years or so a number of diet books, videos and regimes have been marketed advertising miraculous effects. They claim that a dieter can lose more weight than is safe, yet be safe. One has only to read the medical journals to discover how untrue those claims are.

These diets tend to have three things in common: they all restrict fat intake, they all restrict calories, and none of them work. Yes, you will lose some weight but in over ninety-seven per cent of cases it all goes back on again – and usually a bit more besides. So you try another diet, buy another book or join another club – and, of course, spend more money.

Over ninety per cent of the British population has tried dieting at some time or other, and at any one time a third of the adult population is trying to lose weight. The British spend £850 million and Americans spend $33 billion (£25 billion) a year on this quest, so a prosperous slimming industry can be assured of a never-ending income as products and articles promising unattainable goals persuade women (mostly) to attempt the impossible.

Magazine publishers know that many women are so desperate to lose weight that, although they constantly fail, they will try any and every new diet that comes along. Whatever it is, they want to be the first to try it. It is not a new phenomenon: as long ago as 29 March 1957, a 108 kg (17 stone) woman appeared on the British ITV programme *State Your Case for £100*. She said that she wanted the money so that she could attend what she called a 'slimming farm'. She did not get the money. No doubt if she'd had £100 (about two months' wages for the average man in 1957) at the time she would have spent it all on slimming. The mere fact that she appeared on the programme at all in front of millions of viewers demonstrated the strength of her need. So diet after diet is published – all destined to fail, but fail in such a way that they make you need the next one. It becomes an addiction that is created and nurtured by the slimming and food industries for profit.

Slimming clubs and counsellors are only too aware that the modern slimmer will sacrifice anything to lose weight. They set unreasonably low target weights and encourage unreasonably rapid weight loss. Many slimmers find these regimes impossible to resist. Do they work? Only in the short term, and then the weight returns. After losing 64.5 kg (10 stone) in a year and becoming the British 1980 Weight Watcher of the Year, the recipient of this honour said that the experience had changed his life. Suddenly, he was no longer a loser but a success. But the euphoria did not last for long. As soon as he had reached his target weight, the weight he had lost began to return. After a twelve-year struggle, his weight in 1992 was 134 kg (21 stone) – right back where it started. Interviewed on television, he said that the whole weight-loss philosophy was wrong. Slimmers' minds are focused and concentrated on food, when food was the last thing they should be thinking about. He went on to say that his mood now was one of depression, disappointment and a loss of self-esteem, feelings all too common in the long-term slimmer.

Even in specialist hospital obesity clinics, you may not be much better off (although there is the advantage that, as part of the NHS, attendance at one won't cost you anything). An audit of treatments and outcomes was carried out by workers at the Medical Unit, St Bartholomew's Hospital, London, in 1998. They found that only a third of patients lost more than five per cent of their body weight during their treatment phase; forty-three per cent lost between nothing and four per cent; and twenty-five per cent gained weight. Twenty-four per cent of patients reported depressive symptoms and required psychiatric or psychological care or antidepressive drugs.

As some women have realised that low-calorie dieting does not work, they have turned to more drastic measures. They have had their stomachs stapled so that they cannot eat so much; their jaws wired together so that all they can ingest is liquids; their small intestines shortened to reduce the amounts of energy they will absorb; or fat cells removed with liposuction or surgery. These are dangerous and drastic steps which do not always work: one woman who had her jaws wired explained in a TV interview how she liquidised chocolate bars so she could eat them. All these measures seem to achieve in the long run is a lot of pain and suffering followed by a loss of morale and self-esteem when they fail.

Frightening people into cutting down on calories and eating specially prepared, nutritionally poor but expensive 'healthy' or 'slimming' foods meant large profits for the food industry. But anyone who has ever been on a low-calorie diet must know that, in the long run, they simply will not work. Even the medical profession is recognising this truth. Professor Susan Wooley of the University of Cincinnati's College of Medicine and David M. Garner, Director of Research at the Beck Institute for Cognitive Therapy and Research, state:

> The failure of fat people to achieve a goal they seem to want – and to want almost above all else – must now be admitted for what it is: a failure not of those people but of the methods of treatment that are used.

In other words, blaming the overweight for their problem and telling them they are eating too much and must cut down, is simply not good enough. It is the dieticians' advice and the treatment offered that are wrong. Wooley and Garner conclude:

> We should stop offering ineffective treatments aimed at weight loss. Researchers who think they have invented a better mousetrap should test it in controlled research before setting out their bait for the entire population. Only by admitting that our treatments do not work – and showing

that we mean it by refraining from offering them – can we undo a century of recruiting fat people for failure.

There is 'a better mousetrap': presented in this book, which has proved to be very effective and safe ever since its invention over a century ago.

You *can* eat fat and get thin!

Weight control combined with good nutrition need be neither dreary nor difficult. Eat Fat, Get Thin is really not a 'diet' in the way slimmers usually interpret the word. It is only a diet in the sense that everything you eat constitutes your diet, and it is actually the correct way to eat. With Eat Fat, Get Thin:

- you eat naturally
- you eat to enjoy food
- you are in control of your food
- your food does not control you.

It is easy to lose weight – all you need to do is starve. The problem is keeping the weight lost from going back on again. This is where Eat Fat, Get Thin is unlike all the others: you really can stay on this 'diet' for the rest of your life.

If you are overweight, there is little doubt that you will have to change the way you eat. But when you follow Eat Fat, Get Thin you no longer have to count calories consciously. Given the right foods, your body will do that for you automatically, the way it was designed to do naturally.

Eat Fat, Get Thin advocates a diet that does not cut out fats. Although fat has recently had a bad press, until a couple of decades or so ago this would not have been thought odd. Fats are essential for health. Cut them out and you will shorten your life. And, as you will learn, fat actually helps you to slim.

Eat Fat, Get Thin gives you a rare opportunity to hear the other side of the slimming and health debate. It questions low-calorie slimming diets because history, epidemiology and countless scientifically conducted clinical trials have shown that their whole philosophy is wrong. Unlike all other diets,

- Eat Fat, Get Thin does not count calories

- Eat Fat, Get Thin does not cut fats

- Eat Fat, Get Thin does not fail.

I have a number of people successfully losing weight on this diet. A typical one is an overweight civil airline pilot. His wife, also overweight, came to see me and started on this diet in mid-1997. Her husband decided he would join her although he thought that, having to eat the set meals his airline supplied, it would be difficult to do. It was not: he found he merely had to eat more of some things and leave others. After a couple of months his, as well as his wife's, weight had dropped significantly. His reaction was: 'I can't believe this is working; I enjoy it too much.'

The only difficulty I have with Eat Fat, Get Thin is getting people to believe that it can work. Cross that hurdle and your problems are over – for life.

How to use this book

Part 1 explores the theoretical and historical background to the Eat Fat, Get Thin diet, showing how, owing to our genetic inheritance, we need a diet that is high in protein, low in carbohydrate and contains a percentage of animal fats. It explains how the human body processes various types of food, and disproves the current theories that blame fat for the rising incidence of heart disease, for example. It also demonstrates the potential dangers of following the fashionable trends that promote excessive exercise coupled with a high-carbohydrate nutritional regime.

Part 2 sets out the structure of the Eat Fat, Get Thin diet in detail and shows you how to meet your body's requirements on a day-to-day basis. It explains the importance of beginning the day with a good breakfast and contains a number of appetising recipe suggestions for each meal. At the back of the book you will find additional background information, including a glossary, bibliography and comprehensive tables giving the carbohydrate content and glycaemic index of foods.

PART
One

1

The High-Fat Diet Debate

If we do not learn from the past, we remain in the infancy of knowledge.
CICERO

Our story starts with one of the most famous books on obesity ever written. First published in 1863, it went into many editions and continued to be published long after the author's death. A small booklet entitled *Letter on Corpulence Addressed to the Public*, it was written not by a dietician or a doctor but by an undertaker named William Banting. The book was revolutionary and it should have changed Western medical thinking on diet for weight loss for ever.

Undertaker to the rich and famous, William Banting was well regarded in nineteenth-century society. But if he had remained only that, he would probably be remembered today merely as the Duke of Wellington's coffin maker, if at all.

None of Banting's family on either parent's side had any tendency to obesity. Nevertheless it was a condition he dreaded. When he was in his thirties, he started to become overweight and he consulted an eminent surgeon, a kind personal friend, who recommended 'increased bodily exertion before any ordinary daily labours began'. Banting had a heavy boat and lived near the river so he took up rowing the boat for two hours a day. All this did for him, however, was to give him a prodigious appetite. He put on weight and was told to stop.

Banting went into hospital twenty times in as many years for weight reduction. He tried swimming, walking, riding and taking the sea air. He drank 'gallons of physic and liquor potassae', took the spa waters at Leamington, Cheltenham and Harrogate, and tried low-calorie, starvation diets; he took Turkish baths at a rate of up to three a week for a year but lost less than 3 kg (6 lb) in all that time, and had less and less energy.

Discouraged and disillusioned – and still very fat – he gave up. By 1862, at the age of sixty-four, William Banting weighed 91 kg (202 lb or 14 stone 6 lb). He was 1.65 metres (5 foot 5 inches) tall. He says that, although he was of no great weight or size, he:

> could not stoop to tie my shoes, so to speak, nor to attend to the little offices humanity requires without considerable pain and difficulty which only the corpulent can understand. I have been compelled to go downstairs slowly backward to save the jar of increased weight on the knee and ankle joints and have been obliged to puff and blow over every slight exertion, particularly that of going upstairs.

He also had an umbilical rupture, and other bodily ailments. If this were not bad enough, he found that his eyesight was failing and he was becoming increasingly deaf.

In August 1862 Banting consulted a noted Fellow of the Royal College of Surgeons: an ear, nose and throat specialist, Dr William Harvey. It was an historic meeting.

Dr Harvey had recently returned from a symposium in Paris where he had heard Dr Claude Bernard, a renowned physiologist, talk of a new theory about the part the liver played in diabetes. Bernard believed that the liver, as well as secreting bile, also secreted a sugar-like substance that it made from elements of the blood passing through it. This inspired Harvey to research the way in which fats, sugars and starches affect the body.

When Dr Harvey met Banting, he was as much interested by Banting's obesity as by his deafness, for he recognised that the one was the cause of the other, and put him on a diet.

Until that point, Banting's diet had followed this pattern:

> bread and milk for breakfast, or a pint of tea with plenty of milk and sugar, and buttered toast; meat, beer, much bread (of which he had always been fond) and pastry for dinner; a meal of tea similar to breakfast; and generally a fruit tart or bread and milk for supper.

This gave him little comfort and even less sound sleep.

Harvey's advice was to give up bread, butter, milk, sugar, beer and potatoes. These, he told Banting, contained starch and saccharine matter that tended to create fat and were to be avoided altogether.

Banting's immediate thought was that he had very little left to live on. His kind friend soon showed him that really there was ample and within a very few days he derived immense benefit from the plan: it led to an excellent night's rest with six to eight hours' sleep per night.

For each meal, Harvey allowed Banting up to 175 grams (6 oz) of bacon, beef, mutton, venison, kidneys, fish or any form of poultry or game; the 'fruit of any pudding' (he was denied the pastry); any vegetable except potato; and at dinner, two or three glasses of good claret, sherry or Madeira. Banting could drink tea without milk or sugar. Champagne, port and beer were forbidden and he was rationed to 25 grams (1 oz) of toast.

On this diet Banting lost nearly 450 grams (1 lb) per week from August 1862 to August 1863. After thirty-eight weeks, Banting felt better than he had for the last twenty years. By the end of one year, not only had his hearing been restored, he had much more vitality, could exercise freely, had lost 21 kg (46 lb) in weight and 310 mm (12$^{1}/_{4}$ inches) from around his waist. The umbilical rupture was much eased and gave him no anxiety, his sight was restored, and his other bodily ailments had 'passed into the matter of history'.

Banting was delighted. He would have gone through hell to achieve all this but it had not been necessary. Indeed the diet allowed so much food, and it was so easy to maintain, that Banting said of it: 'I can conscientiously assert I never lived so well as under the new plan of dietary, which I should have formerly thought a dangerous, extravagant trespass upon health.' It is obvious from these comments that Banting didn't need the strength of will-power that today's slimmer needs; he found his weight-loss diet very easy to maintain.

Fortunately for us today, in May 1863, after just thirty-eight weeks on his miraculous diet, Banting published and gave away a thousand copies of his now famous *Letter on Corpulence* at his own expense.

The debate begins

The information in Banting's booklet was so contrary to the established doctrine that a howl of protest went up among members of the medical profession. They attacked 'The Banting Diet' on the grounds that it was unscientific, and it became the centre of a bitter controversy.

Dr Harvey was in a difficult position. He had found an effective treatment for obesity but lacked a convincing theory to explain it. He was ridiculed by others in his profession, and his practice began to suffer.

However, the public was impressed. Many desperate, overweight people tried the diet and found that it worked.

To the rescue came a Dr Felix Niemeyer from Stuttgart. By fundamentally altering the basis of the diet, he managed to make it acceptable. The current theory was that carbohydrates and fat burned together in the lungs to produce heat. The two were called 'respiratory foods'. Only these – and not protein – were fattening. Niemeyer, therefore, interpreted 'meat' to mean only lean meat with the fat trimmed off. The altered Banting diet, now a high-protein diet with both carbohydrate and fat restricted, still forms the basis of slimming diets today.

Banting's descriptions of his diet are quite clear, however. Only carbohydrate – sugars and starches – are restricted. Other than the prohibitions against butter and pork (thought to contain too much starch), nowhere is there any instruction to remove the fat from meat and there are no rules about how food should be cooked or how much may be eaten.

Banting, who lived in physical comfort and remained at a normal weight until his death at the age of eighty-one, always maintained that Dr Niemeyer's altered diet was far inferior to the one that had radically changed his life.

Support for the Banting diet

Letter on Corpulence travelled widely. In the 1890s, an American doctor, Helen Densmore, modelled diets on the Banting regime. She tells how she and her patients lost an average 4.5– 6.8 kg (10–15 lb) in the first month on the diet and then 2.7–3.6 kg (6–8 lb) in subsequent months 'by a diet from which bread, cereals and starchy food were excluded'. In 1898 a German doctor, N. Zuntz, reported a case of a man who gained weight on a high-carbohydrate diet and lost weight on a high-fat diet, both of which had similar calorific values. Two American doctors clinically confirmed Zuntz's observation in 1907 with a subject who did uniform amounts of work each day on a bicycle ergometer.

Stefansson and Anderson

In 1906, Dr Vilhjalmur Stefansson spent a winter with the Eskimos of the Canadian Arctic eating a meat and fish diet containing no plant material whatsoever. The usual Eskimo meal consisted of briefly stewed fish washed down with water. It was so different from what Stefansson was used to that at first he was repelled by it. To try to make the fish more palatable, he tried broiling it. This resulted in his becoming weak and dizzy, with other symptoms of malnutrition. Eventually he became so accustomed to the primitive diet that he remained in perfect health and did not get fat.

Some years after his first experience with the Eskimos, Dr Stefansson returned to the Arctic with a colleague, Dr Karsten Anderson, for four years, during which time the two men ate only the meat they could kill and the fish they could catch.

In 1928, Stefansson and Anderson entered Bellevue Hospital, New York, for a controlled experiment into the effects of an all-meat diet on the body. The study showed that there were no deficiency problems; the two men remained perfectly healthy; their bowels remained normal, except that their stools were smaller and did not smell. The absence of starchy and sugary carbohydrates from their diet appeared to have only good effects.

Only when fats were restricted did Stefansson suffer any problems. His intake had varied between 2,000 and 3,100 calories per day and he derived, by choice, an average of eighty per cent of his energy from animal fat and the other twenty per cent from protein.

One interesting finding from a heart disease perspective was that Stefansson's blood cholesterol level *fell* by 1.3

mmol/l while on the all-meat diet, rising again at the end of the study when he resumed a 'normal' diet.

The evidence mounts

- In 1931 Drs D. M. Lyon and D. M. Dunlop of the Royal Infirmary, Edinburgh, conducted a controlled dietary trial using a wide variety of low- and high-calorie diets. On the low-calorie diets, average losses were found to depend on the *carbohydrate content* of the diet. The average weight loss for those on the low-calorie diets was 145 grams per day but those on the *high*-calorie diets lost more, at 157 grams per day. In other words, *the more carbohydrate was eaten, the less weight was lost.*

- In 1944, Dr Blake F. Donaldson carried out a famous experiment at the New York Hospital. Very overweight patients were put on high-fat, low-carbohydrate diets, encouraged to eat as much as they wanted – and *lost weight.*

- After World War II, the E. I. du Pont de Nemours chemical company of America undertook a slimming programme with some of its overweight executives. They were allowed to eat all the untrimmed meat they wanted, with only carbohydrates withheld. The results were spectacular. On the high-calorie diet, they each lost an average *10 kg (22 lb) in three months*, on energy intakes averaging 3,000 calories a day.

- In 1956 Professor Alan Kekwick and Dr Gaston Pawan conducted clinical tests of Banting's diet at the Middlesex Hospital in London. Four 1,000-calorie diets were formulated: ninety per cent carbohydrate; ninety per cent protein; ninety per cent fat; and a normal mixed diet. It became obvious that what a person's diet contained was far more important than the number of calories it contained. Subjects on the high-fat diet lost much more weight than those on the others, while several on the high-carbohydrate diet actually put weight on. In further tests, calorie intakes were *increased* to 2,600 by increasing the amounts of fat and protein, while at the same time the amount of carbohydrate was reduced. This time patients lost weight. There was only one possible explanation: *carbohydrate – sugars and starches – put weight on whereas fats took weight off.*

• Similar findings had been published the previous year by Drs Hausberger and Milstein at Jefferson Medical College in the USA. In their experiments they too demonstrated that *the greater the amount of fat in the diet, the greater the weight loss.* In this test, subjects could eat as much as they liked. The diet which caused by far the greatest weight gain was the one that was practically fat free but high in carbohydrate – similar to those recommended today for weight loss!

These experiments and others, carried out over nearly a century, all showed that *eating fat actually speeds up weight loss*; that for slimming a high-fat, low-carbohydrate diet is best and a high-carbohydrate, low-fat diet is the worst.

Around the turn of the century, doctors devised a simple concept, based on the laws of thermodynamics, likening the body to a tank, into one end of which energy is poured in the form of food. This is then either used up or stored. If you use up more than you pour in, you get thinner and if you pour in more than you use, you get fatter. The theory was easy to understand, made sense, obeyed the laws of physics, and for a while it seemed satisfactory. Dieticians could now say, apparently with scientific backing, that fat people must either be eating too much or working too little.

By the start of the 1914–18 war, however, doubts were creeping in. For instance, diabetes is a defect of carbohydrate metabolism and the treatment for diabetics at that time involved completely depriving them of carbohydrate. In this case, scientists found that the energy input/energy output sums simply did not add up.

By the early 1920s, interest in the theory was renewed. It was found to be impossible to measure the total amount of water in a person at any one time. Therefore, water retention or loss was said to account for any discrepancy in the balance between energy input/output and excess weight. It was decades before this convenient theory was disproved.

In the 1950s, isotope techniques were developed which allowed more accurate measurement of body fat turnover. In addition, it was demonstrated that different foods could alter the amounts of body fat; and that body fat could also be affected by certain responsive glands – the adrenal, thyroid and pituitary glands – even when energy intake was constant.

The flaws exposed

The fact that high-energy diets are more effective for reducing weight may seem puzzling, and it has proved very difficult for dieticians and doctors to accept, because it appears to challenge the laws of thermodynamics. But there are flaws in this theory. To grasp them, we need to go over some basic facts.

The calorie is a unit of heat. The way the energy content of a food is determined is by burning it in a device called a 'bomb calorimeter' and measuring the amount of heat it gives off.

A gram of carbohydrate gives an energy value of 4.2 calories, or more correctly kilocalories (kcals). A gram of protein gives 5.25 kcals. This time, however, one calorie is deducted because a gram of protein does not oxidise readily, it gives rise to urea and other products which must be subtracted. That gives a final figure for protein of 4.25 kcals. Burning a gram of fat in the bomb calorimeter gives 9.2 kcals.

These figures are then rounded to the nearest whole number – 4, 4 and 9 respectively – and are used in calorie charts to indicate the energy values of foodstuffs and, thus, to allow slimmers to measure their food intake.

But there are two basic flaws in using these figures to determine the amounts of food we should eat:

1. The more obvious flaw in the argument is that our bodies do not burn foods in the same way that they are burned in a bomb calorimeter. If they did, we would glow in the dark. The digestive process is quite inefficient. The chemical process whereby blood sugar is oxidised to provide energy produces carbon dioxide. About half is exhaled as carbon dioxide, the other half is excreted in sweat, urine and faeces as energy-containing molecules, the energy values of which must be deducted from the original food intake. All of these vary. For example, eating a lot of fat forms ketones, which can be found in urine. The value of a gram of ketones derived from fat is roughly four calories. So, in this case, nearly half the energy from the fat is lost.

2. The second and more important flaw in the argument is that the body does not use all its food to provide energy. The primary function of dietary proteins, for example, is body cell manufacture and repair: making skin, blood, hair and finger- and toe-nails, etc. The amount of protein needed for this purpose is generally accepted to be about one gram per kilogram of lean body weight. As meats contain approximately 23 grams of protein per 100 grams, a person weighing, say, 70 kg (11 stone) needs to eat about 300 g (11 oz) of meat, or its equivalent, every day just to supply his basic protein needs. Even eating this volume of lean chicken would

provide some 465 calories. These calories are not used to supply energy, they contribute nothing to the body's calorie needs and so must be deducted if you are counting calories.

Much of the fat we eat is also used to provide materials used by the body in processes other than the production of energy: the manufacture of bile acids and hormones, the essential fatty acids for the brain and nervous system, and so on. All these must be deducted as well. Thus trying to determine, from food intake and energy expenditure alone, how much excess energy your body will store as fat will give a completely wrong answer. However, these other factors cannot be measured. Calorie-counting, which is the foundation of practically every modern slimming diet, is a complete waste of time.

The dietician's ally

By the late 1950s, as the result of one misrepresented study, fat began to be suspected of contributing to the rising incidence of coronary heart disease in Western countries. Banting's low-carbohydrate, high-fat, diet began to go out of fashion.

In 1983 and 1984, two British committees, the National Advisory Committee for Nutrition Education (NACNE) and the Committee on the Medical Aspects of Food Policy (COMA), published reports which recommended that dietary fats be reduced to prevent the growing problem of heart disease.

Whether from animal or vegetable sources, fats and proteins tend to go together. It is difficult to reduce fat intake, therefore, without also reducing protein intake. Foods high in protein alone are also more expensive. Dieticians now appeared to have justification for recommending a change to carbohydrates: indeed it was the only food group left which they could recommend.

Carbohydrates have the advantage that they contain the fewest calories and provide the least energy. The recommendation to reduce fat intake for 'health' reasons, coupled with a recommendation that we should be eating more carbohydrates, turned slimming diets into the total opposite of what all the evidence says they should be.

Which is why, in the 1990s, at a time when most of us are dieting, are eating fewer calories and less fat, and taking more exercise than ever before in our history, we are getting fatter than ever before in our history.

The paradox resolved

For nearly a century and a half, it has been shown beyond doubt that eating a high-energy diet can assist weight loss. The answer to this apparent paradox is the clue to achieving and maintaining a normal weight.

Glycogen, a form of starch, is the principal form in which carbohydrate is stored in the body. The process that converts the blood sugar, glucose, into glycogen is called *glycogenesis*. Eating foods that are highly glycogenic, which means they are easily converted into starch, will lead to weight gain. In 1932, Drs Lyon and Dunlop noticed that weight loss appeared to be inversely proportional to the amount of glycogenic foods in the diet. Dr Albert Pennington points out that, whereas carbohydrate is one hundred per cent glycogenic and protein is fifty-eight per cent glycogenic, fat is only ten per cent glycogenic.* Thus fat is the least likely to put weight on, and the best at getting weight off.

---

* A more modern version of this principle, the glycaemic index of foodstuffs, is discussed on pages 197–205.

2

It's In Our Genes

As we have seen, studies show that eating an unrestricted diet, composed mainly of proteins and fats, helps in the battle of the bulge; that cutting calories, and, particularly, cutting fats, does not. But fats contain the most energy, so how can this be so? The answer lies in the way our bodies have evolved to deal with the different foods.

Our natural diet

Books written by nutritionists and dieticians tend to be contradictory, often reflecting current fads. As they cannot all be right, how are we to determine what is our natural diet?

The answer lies in our past. Not the immediate past: the way we live now is based on advanced agriculture and the domestication of plants and animals, recent innovations to which we cannot yet have become adapted. To determine what foods are likely to make up a natural diet for mankind as a species, we must look further back, at our evolutionary history. For the food we are genetically programmed to eat is determined by what has been coded in our genes over millions of years.

We can trace human evolution from remains and artefacts of early hominids found in Africa and other parts of the world dated as long as four million years ago; we have fossilised bone records of both our hominid ancestors and of animals; we have stone tools and implements that must have been used for killing and cutting flesh or for grinding plants; we even have hominid faeces. These findings have led to a great deal of speculation about our diet. Are we a carnivorous, omnivorous or a herbivorous species?

We call our ancestors and the various modern primitive tribes 'hunter-gatherers'. In the world today, some tribes live exclusively on meat and fish; others live largely on fruit, nuts and roots, although meat is also highly prized; still more live without eating anything derived from animal sources. It is obvious, therefore, that as a species we can survive on a wide variety of foods. But which, if any, is the diet that we have evolved to eat?

Three possible combinations of diet can be considered for early humans:

1. wholly carnivorous, hunting and killing animals;

2. omnivorous, eating a mixed diet of both animal and plant origin;

3. herbivorous, i.e. vegetarians eating no meat at all.

The vegetarian hypothesis explored

The vegetarian hypothesis has it that early humans were wholly dependent on plant foods and that meat never played an important part in our evolution. It is a hypothesis that has fervent support in the USA and it is gaining ground in Britain and other developed countries.

In our hunt for an answer, the first evidence to consider lies in the fossil sites of Africa, widely accepted as our birthplace. Here, where hominid remains are found, so also are animal bones – sometimes in their thousands. If those hominids were not meat-eaters, why is that? Second, although many modern hunting tribes do eat plants, they have fire. There were very few plant foods with sufficient calorific value that our prehistoric ancestors could have digested without fire. There were fruits, of course, but there is not one prehistoric site in all Africa that indicates forests extensive enough to have supplied sufficient fruit to meet the needs of its inhabitants There is agreement that our ancestors did not dwell in forests at all but on the savannah, where there were vast plains of grass. However, grass is of no value whatsoever to the human digestive system. Even to live off the fleshier leaves would require the much more highly specialised digestive systems found in other primates, such as gorillas.

The walls of all plant cells are made of cellulose, a form of dietary fibre. There is no enzyme in the human digestive system that will break it down. And with the cell walls intact, the nutrients in the cells cannot be digested. Passing unaffected straight through the gut, they would be ejected as waste.

Neither is it likely that the seeds of the savannah grasses could have supplied early humans with the energy they required. Seeds are naturally indigestible, designed to pass through an animal's body, to be defecated and take root elsewhere. There are two means whereby seeds can be made digestible: cooking and grinding. Seeds could have been pounded to break down the plant cell walls, but no archaeologist has ever found a Stone Age tool suited to this task.

If seeds had been ground down by chewing, fossilised teeth would show a great deal more wear than they do; in addition, a very large proportion of the seeds would have escaped and, passing through the body undigested, ended up in the faeces. Fossilised hominid faeces, known as coprolites, have been studied in detail and almost none contain any plant material.

Homo erectus began to appreciate the value of fire around 350,000 years ago. If our ancestors had started cooking grains then, we could have evolved and adapted to them by now. To process grains and other seeds, you need either to crush them and make the flour into a paste, or a container of some sort to cook them in. The absence of suitable tools makes the former unlikely, and the latter can be discounted because the oldest known pot is just 6,800 years old. (In evolutionary terms, that was only yesterday.)

Cooking also requires a controlled fire. Although hearths have been discovered that are 100,000 years old, these are very rare. European Neanderthal coprolites dating from around 50,000 years ago, before fire was used, contain no plant material. It was not until the Cro-Magnon colonisation of Europe, some 35,000 years ago, that hearths became universal. Even then the evidence suggests that they were not used for cooking plants but merely for warmth. At the time, Europe was in the grip of a succession of ice ages. For some 70,000 years there were long, cold winters and short, cool summers. Cro-Magnon man and his Eurasian ancestors cannot have been plant-eaters then – for most of the year there weren't any plants! They ate meat or died. And they ate that meat raw.

The evidence that we could not be a vegetarian species was already overwhelming and in 1972 the publication of two independent investigations confirmed this. They concerned fats.

About half our brain and nervous system is composed of complicated, long-chain, fatty acid molecules, which are also used by the walls of our blood vessels. Without them we cannot develop normally. These fatty acids do not occur in plants, although fatty acids in a simpler form do. This is where the plant-eating herbivores come in. Over the year, they convert the simple fatty acids found in grasses and seeds into intermediate, more complicated forms. By eating the herbivores we can convert the herbivore's store of the less complex fatty acids into the ones we need.

Our brain is considerably larger than that of any ape. Looking back at the fossil records from early hominids to modern man, we see a remarkable increase in brain size. This expansion could not have happened without large quantities of the right kinds of fatty acids. It would never have occurred if our ancestors had not eaten meat. Human breast milk contains the fatty acids needed for large brain development, cow's milk does not. It is no coincidence that, in relative terms, our brain is some fifty times the size of a cow's.

The vegetarian may also be dismayed to learn that while soy bean is rich in complete protein, and grains and nuts also combine to provide complete proteins, none contains the fats that are essential for proper brain development.

We cannot be a vegetarian species. From at least the time of *Homo erectus* some 500,000 years ago, we must have lived on and adapted to a diet composed almost exclusively of meat.

What early humans really ate

Early man hunted and ate meat primarily but, if meat were in short supply, would eat almost anything – so long as it did not require cooking. This still precluded some of the roots and most of the seeds we eat today.

We also have a sense of taste for sweet things, a tendency we would not have developed if it served no function. So fruit must have formed part of our ancestors' diet. But fruit contains little or no protein, and protein on a daily basis is essential for health. Out of necessity they must have obtained protein from nuts. When times were good, their diet was high in animal protein and fat, supplemented with wild fruit; only during lean times did it include other foods of vegetable origin. Therefore our ideal diet, the one we have evolved and adapted to, must be one which is high in proteins and fats, and low in carbohydrates.

Agriculture and the first diet revolution

It was not until the last ice age came to an end about 10,000 years ago and the ice receded, that there was sufficient surplus food for some to be stored; some previously nomadic tribes were able to develop stable settlements. The cultivation of wild seeds began. From these are derived the cereals we know today, such as wheat, barley, maize, and rice. These had the advantage that they did not deteriorate readily and could be stored for long periods against winter famines. Cooking solved the problem of their indigestibility.

This development caused a dramatic change in man's lifestyle. The capacity to store controlled quantities of higher-energy starches meant that their numbers could grow. And as numbers grew, it became more difficult to maintain food supplies through hunting alone. Thus our ancestors' basic diet changed from a high protein/fat diet to one containing more starchy carbohydrates.

There is no evidence of nutritional diseases before the invention of agriculture. After it, there is. Cereals that became the modern staples, together with root crops which began to be cultivated, are all relatively deficient in protein, vitamins and several minerals, notably iron and calcium. Additionally, all cereals contain a substance called phytate that binds with some minerals and other nutrients and reduces the ability of the body to absorb them. As a consequence, the coming of agriculture gave rise to nutritional diseases such as rickets, pellagra, dental caries, beriberi, obesity, allergies and cancers: the so-called 'diseases of civilisation'.

The industrial revolution and the second diet revolution

About 200 years ago the industrial revolution heralded a second dietary revolution which had two powerful but opposite effects on our health. Industrialised countries like Britain, with their increased wealth, no longer had to rely on home-produced, seasonally dependent foods: they could import what they wanted. They could look forward to going through life without ever being hungry. However, there were adverse effects.

Many of the imported foods were unnatural to those eating them. New fruits tasted nice and, as a consequence, people changed from eating what they needed to eating what they liked. Unaided by previous experience, the human autonomic nervous system had never learned when to stop.

As time went by, science made possible the production of synthetic foods that had the appearance, texture and taste of the real thing, but with few of the proteins and vitamins. Sugar became easy and cheap to produce, leading to a thirty-fold increase in its consumption. The industrial revolution, therefore, was something of a double-edged sword: on the one hand it gave people a wider range of food than had ever before been possible, on the other, diabetes, peptic ulcers, heart disease were added to the list of new diseases. In the late twentieth century the pace at which our diet has become increasingly unnatural has quickened.

Our early ancestors' food, whether from animal or vegetable sources, was eaten raw. Now cooking food has become a way of life. Cooking is the only means of breaking down starches so that we can digest them. As a consequence, cereals and many other starchy vegetables need not only to be cooked, but to be well cooked, before they can be digested. Cooking can cause problems. It destroys some nutrients: vitamin C is a notable example. Thus nutrients that might be present when food is 'natural' are lost and their correct balance may also be lost.

Food has radically changed and in a time span much too short for us to have evolved and adapted to it. This is particularly so in the case of carbohydrates.

Unnatural processing

A number of vegetable-based foods are processed to such a high degree that nothing but pure carbohydrate is left. The obvious example is white granulated sugar. Sugar cane and sugar beet contain a significant proportion of protein, vitamins, minerals and fibre. But all these are lost during processing. The end product is a pure, concentrated carbohydrate: a chemical called sucrose. For their metabolism, all carbohydrates require vitamins. These too are lost in the processing of sugar, so that when sugar is eaten, it uses up some of the body's store of these vitamins. Also lost are other nutrients. In a similar way, cereals – wheat, rice, barley and oats – are selectively bred and today, genetically modified, to increase their yield of starch. It is this concentration that is so unnatural.

Protein has not undergone the same process, as it is relatively expensive, and nor have fats, as they are concentrated naturally.

The concentration of carbohydrate allowed a dramatic and rapid increase in its consumption. Annual sugar consumption in Britain in the middle of the eighteenth century was less than 2 kg (4 lb) per person; today it is more than 60 kg (130 lb).

The same is true of cereals. Many packaged foods today contain substances with such names as 'modified starch' or 'maltodextrin'. These too are highly concentrated carbohydrates, in this case cereal starch. These sugars and starches are added to make foods cheaper or more attractive, or to create larger profits for the manufacturers. They have detrimental effects on large sections of the population. Our bodies' natural nutrient-requirement signal, the appetite, has not evolved to cope with such unnatural foods. It knows when to stop us eating meat, but not when to stop us eating chocolate bars and cakes. It is also much easier to eat modern white bread than the stodgy, pre-industrial revolution bread.

Food and disease

A study by Drs W. S. McClellan and E. F. Du Bois found that the Eskimos in Baffin Island and Greenland living on a diet composed almost entirely of meat and fish and eating no starchy or sugary foods were almost completely free from disease. This was not the case with the Labrador Eskimos, who lived on preserved foods, dried potatoes, flour, canned foods and cereals. Among them the diseases of 'civilisation' were rife.

A comparison between the Maasai tribes of East Africa, who live alongside the Kikuyu, shows a similar pattern. The Maasai, when wholly carnivorous, drinking only the blood and milk of their cattle, were tall, healthy, long-lived and slim. The Kikuyu, when wholly vegetarian, were stunted, diseased, short-lived and pot-bellied. Over the last few decades, the Kikuyu have started to eat meat, and their health has improved. Since 1960 the Maasai diet has also changed, but in the opposite direction. They are now eating less blood and milk, replacing them with maize and beans. Their health has deteriorated. The same is true of every tribe that has had contact with Western civilisation.

Sugar and starch

All slimmers know that sugar, above all else, is fattening.
Every diet yet devised counsels, quite rightly, against
eating sugar. At the same time, many modern dieticians
also tell dieters that they should eat more starchy foods:
bread, pasta or potatoes. However, it doesn't matter
whether you eat sugar and jam or pasta, bread, and
breakfast cereals; the digestion makes no distinction. *All*
the carbohydrates you eat are destined to be converted and
enter your bloodstream as the blood sugar, glucose.

Refined, concentrated sugars and starches are used
widely in pre-packed convenience foods. On packaged
foods, the sugar content is frequently obscured by the
manufacturers – sugar contents being variously described
as sucrose, fructose, glucose, maltose or dextrose. But
bread, pasta, rice, and other cereals, are all high in
concentrated starches. And, from a slimming point of
view, these may actually be worse than sugar because,
during digestion, they produce even higher levels of
calories.

The importance of blood sugar levels

The cause of obesity problems in the West is too high an
intake of sugar and other sweet or starchy foods. When the
body's energy and blood sugar levels are low, it signals the
need to eat via the feeling of hunger. Then, if we are
sensible, we eat a meal composed of food items which are
natural to us and which are digested and absorbed at
different rates. This way energy is released continuously
over the period to the next meal. When eaten,
carbohydrates are digested and absorbed quickly, within
minutes; proteins are digested more slowly and fats are
digested last. If we eat the three in the correct proportions,
there will be no problems. If the meal is too high in

carbohydrates, however, blood sugar levels rise rapidly. This blood sugar is metered in the brain by the hypothalamus. When blood sugar levels get too high, the hypothalamus stimulates the pancreas to produce insulin. The insulin converts the excess glucose for storage and reduces the level in the blood. But there is a time lag. By the time the pancreas finds that the blood sugar level has dropped sufficiently, it has produced more than enough insulin to reduce those high blood sugar levels. Blood sugar is driven down to a *low* level, making us feel hungry again. The effect is known as 'reactive hypoglycaemia'. So we eat more – and tend to snack on sweets! It is a vicious circle. We feel hungry even though we eat more, and become run down and depressed. In the mean time the excesses have been converted to fat for storage and we have gained weight.

The answer is to eat *less* carbohydrate so that the blood sugar level does not fluctuate so violently, and eat *more* fat. Because it takes a long time to digest, fat not only prevents those violent fluctuations in blood sugar levels, it gives a feeling of satiety, which stops that feeling of hunger.

As you will have realised, it is not just people wanting to lose weight who should beware of overeating carbohydrates. Apart from making us overweight, a number of other disorders are caused or exacerbated by too high an intake of sugars and starches – environmental diseases from diabetes and heart disease to decayed teeth and fatigue. It even makes us more susceptible to viral diseases such as the common cold.

The cholesterol theory has it that blocked arteries prevent oxygen from reaching the heart muscle, but the majority of people who die of heart disease *do not have blocked coronary arteries*. The blocked artery hypothesis cannot account for this. The oxygen used in muscles to oxidise glucose is only half the equation. Low utilisation of glucose by the heart muscle may be due not to lack of oxygen but to low blood glucose levels. And *low* blood glucose levels are caused by a *high*-carbohydrate diet.

Triglycerides are neutral fats found at high levels in many heart disease cases. Eating too much fat is usually blamed, but blood triglyceride levels have been shown to be proportional not to fat intake but to carbohydrate intake. Platelets, the agents which make blood clot when we are cut, also tend to clump together on a diet high in sugars and refined starches. It has been shown that a diet that contains a large proportion of carbohydrate can cause blood clots and reduce the flow of blood to the extremities. If such a clot reaches the heart, it can cause a blockage in a coronary artery. The best way to reduce the risk of a blood clot and, thus, a heart attack is, again, to reduce your carbohydrate intake. In the next chapter I look more closely at research into heart disease.

One aspect of sugar must be taken into account: sugar is addictive. Although other starchy foods may have a greater immediate effect on blood sugar levels than sugar, you are not likely to yearn after, say, a parsnip. But sugar, and foods that contain it in large quantity, are craved. To ensure that you become addicted and your craving is maintained, food manufacturers now put sugar in just about everything that comes in a packet, tin or bottle – just look at the labels even on tinned meat, for example, and try to find one that does not contain sugar.

A large part of learning to eat for health and to remain slim is concerned with beating the sugar habit. When you can walk past the sweets at a checkout without the desire to buy some, you will be cured. It will take a time, but it is well worth it.

Artificial sweeteners

There is some debate about the role of the artificial sweeteners as used by slimmers. Saccharine and aspartame contain no calories. So, on the face of it, they appear to be an ideal substitute for those people with a sweet tooth who cannot give up sugar. But there are two problems with them:

1. A great deal has been said in the media about artificial sweeteners hampering weight loss. The suggestion is that the pancreas may start to produce insulin for the purpose of reducing blood glucose levels before those levels are elevated, merely in response to a sweet stimulus. Thus eating a calorie-free sweetener can trigger the production of insulin. However, as no glucose enters the bloodstream, glucose already there is removed for storage as fat, blood glucose levels are driven down and the result is hunger and increased food intake.

2. Whether or not the above is correct, it is true that eating foods containing artificial or any other kind of sweeteners maintains the taste for oversweetened foods. It is much better to reduce your use of *all* sweeteners gradually until the natural sweetness of foods tastes right for you. The sweetness to aim for is the natural sweetness found in fruit.

. . . and colds

Colds are looked upon as a fact of life -- everyone gets them and they are not regarded as being serious. But this perception may be incorrect. In 1954, the *British Medical Journal* published an article showing that respiratory infections, particularly colds, were the most common irritating and aggravating factors in congestive heart failure. In two studies of incidences of heart failure, more than half the patients had some form of respiratory infection and a direct correlation was found between the frequent occurrence of heart failure and 'even minor colds'. Colds can be deadly.

The role of refined carbohydrates in respiratory problems was demonstrated dramatically in a study comparing the Kikuyu and Maasai tribes. The Kikuyu, living mainly on cereals, had a mortality from bronchitis and pneumonia which was ten times higher than that of the meat-eating Maasai. A similar comparison carried out at a girls' boarding-school found the same: researchers demonstrated that the incidence of colds among the girls was directly related to the amount of sugar each consumed. Their evidence showed that the girls who drank fizzy drinks and ate sweets and other refined carbohydrates suffered many more respiratory problems and colds than girls who did not. The advice given to reduce the likelihood of getting a cold was to cut out sugar and eat no bread or other products that contain either wheat or rye.

Summary

What we are advised to eat today is far removed from the diet to which we are naturally adapted, and are genetically programmed to eat. Dieticians tell us to eat more bread, pasta, fruit and vegetables. The first two of these are high in refined carbohydrates. For the most part, these are the sources of the carbohydrates in our diets which cause the damage listed above. Things like sugar, sticky sweets, soft drinks, pasta, cakes and white bread are the main culprits. But others that may be harmful in sufficient quantity include dried fruits, such as raisins, and the starchier root vegetables. Cooked, refined carbohydrate foods are worse than raw. Green vegetables, which are generally low in carbohydrates, cooked or uncooked, present no problems.

There is no evidence that proteins are fattening or in any other way harmful, and no convincing evidence that fats from animal sources are either. We may need some carbohydrate in our diet – the evidence one way or the other is unconvincing – but certainly not in large quantities, and not in the form in which most carbohydrate is ingested today.

The best place to get the carbohydrate part of your diet is the greengrocer's shop – not at the baker's or the grocer's – and certainly not at the confectioner's.

3
Eat Less, Weigh More!

He that lives upon hope will die fasting.
BENJAMIN FRANKLIN.

It is simplistic to claim that people get fat because they eat too much, although if you become overweight it is because you have consumed more energy than you have used. To understand obesity, you first need some knowledge of what happens to food and how the body metabolises and regulates energy.

Your body gets its energy from the foods – carbohydrates, proteins and fats – that you eat. Digestion breaks up foods into their constituent compounds. These are then utilised as they are or rebuilt to be used in all your body's processes.

To keep your heart beating, your body warm, your muscles working, and all the other processes going on requires a constant supply of energy (fuel). As you cannot be eating twenty-four hours a day, your body ensures that energy is available at all times by storing it in several forms: as glucose in the blood, which is the most readily available; as glycogen, a form of starch, stored in muscles; as lean tissue; and as fat.

Muscles burn carbohydrate, in the form of glucose, and fat for energy; the brain uses only glucose. If you use up more energy than you take in, your store of glycogen is used first and when that is exhausted body fat and lean tissue are cannibalised to provide the energy required.

Proteins

Proteins are essential to the body, providing the material from which body cells are made and repaired. Proteins are composed of chains of amino-acids. There are hundreds of these in nature. Our bodies use around twenty, which can be arranged in an almost infinite number of ways. Amino-acids are usually split into two groups: *essential* and *non-essential*. The essential amino-acids are those that the body cannot make for itself and which must be present in food. There are eight of them. If a protein contains the eight essential amino-acids, in the correct proportions, it is called a *complete protein*; if it does not, it is said to be an *incomplete protein*.

Complete proteins are found in meat, fish, eggs, dairy products and soy bean. Animal proteins, which are complete, have a high biological value for man. As we are part of the animal kingdom and composed of similar material to other animals, we can use animal proteins with the minimum of waste.

Sources of *incomplete proteins* are cereals, nuts, seeds and legumes. Proportions of amino-acids in any one of these types of vegetable food, with the exception of soy bean, differ markedly from those we need. Maize is deficient in tryptophan, wheat is low in lysine and legumes are low in methionine. Proteins from these vegetable sources are said to be 'of low biological value'. It is necessary, therefore, to combine several vegetable protein sources, fairly accurately, to ensure that the body receives the right amino-acid mixture.

In practical terms, it is not too difficult to combine vegetables to meet our bodies' protein requirements. In these circumstances, the real advantage of meat over the vegetables is their associated nutrients: vitamin B_{12}, vitamin D, iron, calcium and the more complex fatty acids.

As far as weight loss is concerned there is one other advantage to getting your proteins from animal sources: combining the various sources of incomplete proteins to supply all the essential amino-acids on a vegetarian diet could lead to a high intake of carbohydrates.

Your body needs proteins continually but it cannot store them in any quantity. Therefore you should eat proteins regularly on a daily basis, and at the same meal, in quantities proportional to your size. But they must be complete proteins: if only one of the essential amino-acids is missing, the cell rebuilding process will abort.

Carbohydrates

Carbohydrates provide only energy. They have none of the essential components that the body needs to build or repair its tissues. A person fed only carbohydrates would starve to death no matter how much he ate. His body would break down muscle and other body proteins in an attempt to keep the essential organs functioning. At the same time he would put on weight while he died, as the carbohydrate surplus was stored as body fat. Just as we store energy as fat, so plants store energy as starch and sugar. Thus foods of vegetable origin are rich in these carbohydrates.

Daily protein requirements

A 'balanced' diet is simply one that provides all the nutrients your body needs in sufficient quantity to prevent deficiencies from occurring. Nutrients such as vitamins and minerals, which are required in small quantities, can all be met on a restricted-calorie diet because supplementary pills can be taken. However, where your body needs large amounts of a particular nutrient, it is not so easy.

Your body needs complete proteins every day, and with proteins come calories. The average woman could realistically get her protein needs from the foods in the table below. (Although I do not advocate a low-fat diet, I have deliberately made this example typical of the kinds of foods slimmers are advised to eat to illustrate realistically the extent of the danger of malnutrition if you cut calories too much.)

EXAMPLE OF MINIMUM DAILY PROTEIN REQUIREMENTS

	Protein (grams)	Calories
125 grams lean meat	30	250
1 egg	6	75
50 grams cottage cheese	12	185
570 ml (1 pint) semi-skimmed milk	16	275
2 slices bread	4	120
Total	68	905

Men need about 25 to 50 grams more meat or another egg.

Your body also needs a certain amount of fat, if only to supply the essential fatty acids needed for proper brain function, you must eat at least 15 grams of these per day. That adds another 135 calories, but as the foods in the examples all contain these fats, the calories they contain are already included.

It is clear that a 1,000-calorie diet, for instance, must be composed almost exclusively of foods which are very high in protein and fats if you are to take in the *minimum* amount of these nutrients to be healthy. Therefore a crash diet supplying, say, 500 calories a day must be harmful to health. The low-fat, high-carbohydrate slimming diets advocated today will inevitably be dangerously deficient in protein.

The importance of fat

The science of nutrition is highly complex and little is known about the vital part that fat plays in our health and wellbeing. Nutrients interact: a deficiency of one can have a profound effect on the metabolism of others. Today, a lack of dietary fat probably causes a wider range of abnormalities than deficiencies of any other single nutrient.

Fat provides more than twice as much energy as carbohydrate, and also contains lipids used in the brain and nervous system, without which we become irritable and aggressive; sterols, precursors of a number of hormones (including the sex hormones); and the fat-soluble vitamins A, D, E and K. These vitamins can be found in other foods, but without the presence of dietary fat, the body cannot metabolise them.

Fat has a high calorific value, which is why all modern low-calorie diets restrict fats, but this can be dangerous and self-defeating. Restriction of dietary fat causes a range of problems including dry skin and eczema; damage to ovaries in females; infertility in males; kidney damage and weight gain through water retention in the body. When there is little or no fat in the gut, there is nothing to stimulate the production of bile, the gall-bladder is not emptied and the bile is held in reserve. This leads to the formation of gallstones. If a fat-free diet is continued for a long time, the gall-bladder – a necessary part of the digestive system – may atrophy.

Malabsorption of the fat-soluble vitamins A, D, E and K has consequences for yet more nutrients. If vitamin D and fat are not present in the intestine, for example, calcium is not absorbed. For a woman, whose chance of suffering from osteoporosis is high, this is an important consideration. Slimmers are usually told to drink skimmed milk. This has the advantage, they are told, that it contains more calcium than full-cream milk. This is true, but skimmed milk does not contain fat. As a consequence, only about five per cent of the calcium in skimmed milk is absorbed, compared to around fifty per cent from full-cream milk. This small absorption of calcium is reduced still further if the skimmed milk is eaten with a bran-laden breakfast cereal. Calcium-enriched milk sold in supermarkets may seem worth the extra expense but it is invariably calcium-enriched *skimmed* milk and, without the cream, all that extra calcium is simply excreted.

Fat is best:

- All body cells require a continuous supply of various fatty acids. If insufficient are supplied from food, the body tries to make them from sugar. This causes blood sugar levels to fall, you feel very hungry and eat more, generally of the wrong things – and gain weight.

- Fat also has a satiety value: it takes longer to digest and stops you feeling hungry. Eat a hundred calories less fat at a meal and you will probably feel hungry so quickly that you will eat three times as many calories – in the form of sugary or starchy foods, because they are convenient.

- It seems that the gut's nutrient-measuring system works so well with fat that it is difficult, if not impossible, to eat too much of it. Try and you develop an aversion to it. But, for the same reason, eating fat stops you eating too much in total. If your body needs 10 grams of fat, your appetite will not be satisfied until you have consumed that 10 grams of fat. If you eat those 10 grams as 25 grams (1 oz) of Cheddar cheese, you will take in about 125 calories. If you eat them as wholemeal bread thinly spread with a very low-fat spread, you will need to eat eight slices – a total of about 500 calories!

Fat improves performance

Athletes, like the rest of us, are usually told to eat a diet high in carbohydrates and low in fats. The theory that this will increase their performance was not confirmed in a dietary study published in 1994. Using three diets: normal, high-fat and high-carbohydrate, the study showed that the high-carbohydrate diet increased performance by an average ten per cent over a normal mixed diet. Not bad, you might think, but the high-fat diet increased performance by a massive thirty-three per cent. The authors conclude that restriction of dietary fat may be detrimental to endurance performance. So, once again, fat is best.

Set point weight

The set point is a natural weight, specific to you, which your body will try to maintain at all costs. It has been found that if lean people are forced to overeat so that they put on weight, as soon as they return to a normal eating pattern, their weight returns to where it started – their set point. Similarly when overweight people go on a low-calorie diet, their bodies try desperately to maintain the higher, set point weight. And, for this reason, as soon as the diet finishes, their bodies use the opportunity to put weight back on – to return to the set point weight. This is another reason that low-calorie dieting is doomed to failure.

Dr Xavier Pi-Sunyer, Director of the Obesity Research Center, St Luke's-Roosevelt Hospital, New York, is convinced that a person's set point works only one way:

upward. He explains that the body tends to allow weight gain without adjustment, but if a person's weight remains at the higher weight for a while, the new higher weight becomes the set point and the body will do its utmost to maintain it.

There is a survival advantage in this. Regularly, throughout human history, food has been in short supply, during the winter months and in the ice ages, for example. We do not hibernate as some animals do, but during our evolution we too developed the ability to store energy against hard times. Those who stored the most had the best chance of surviving a protracted period of relative starvation. We still have that ability, but we now live in a time when there is anything but a food shortage.

Energy regulation systems

Eat only as many calories as your body uses, dieticians tell us. How can this be done? It is impossible to measure by mental arithmetic your energy input to the nearest calorie (or kilojoule) and tailor your workload to use up exactly the same amount as you put in. But your body can.

The systems which regulate food input and energy output are complex but completely self-regulating and extremely accurate. Your body knows exactly how much of any particular nutrient it needs and, if you are aware of it, it will tell you.

The control systems may be divided into two: those which regulate energy input and those which regulate energy output, the two working together to achieve a balance.

Energy intake controls

On the energy intake side, the controls are hunger and appetite. Through appetite the body tells you what combination of proteins, fats, carbohydrates and other nutrients to eat. Without hunger you would not know when to eat and without appetite you would not know what and how much to eat. These are the signals with which your body communicates with you. They measure and time your body's needs very precisely. If these signals are not heeded, those needs are not met and permanent damage can result.

As food is eaten, sensors in the upper gut assess its nutritional appropriateness and set up a chain of electro-chemical reactions involving the gut opiates, chemical messengers that are similar to morphine in their properties but much stronger. Most are in the intestinal nerve cells, others in the hypothalamus. The opiates control hunger and appetite. As each nutrient is supplied, the appetite for it diminishes until, eventually, the appetite for it is satisfied and 'switches off'. When all our energy needs are met, we no longer feel hungry and we (should) stop eating.

The opiates work extremely efficiently with fats and proteins, but they hardly appear to work at all with carbohydrates. You will find that you cannot eat too much fat. You may like butter or cream but try to eat a lot of either and you will soon develop an aversion to it. Try a little experiment with two items of food that you like, one a sweet carbohydrate food such as toffees, the other one of fat, such as butter. You will find that you will be able to eat the toffees until they 'come out of your ears'. Try the same with butter, however, and you probably won't get beyond the second teaspoon before you begin to go off it. Your body is telling you it has had enough. Disregard this signal and you will probably be sick. On the other hand, it is all too easy to eat too many sweets and other refined carbohydrates such as bread and pasta.

It is possible, however, to fool the body to some extent. Andrew Prentice and Susan Jebb of the Medical Research

Council's Dunn Clinical Nutrition Centre suggest that adding sugar to fatty foods can allow you to eat more fat by disguising it and making the fat more palatable. They point out that studies have already been done which showed a reciprocal relation between fat and sugar intake. This is particularly true when fat is combined with sugar and starch in such confections as cakes and chocolates. These are the mixtures that are fattening. The foods which are the major natural contributors to fat intake – meat, fat spreads and oils, dairy products, eggs and fish – are not combined to any great extent with sugar, and are not fattening.

Brown fat cells

The body's use of energy, the output side of the body's energy balance, is controlled by our brown fat. Although mainly located in the upper back, there are clusters of brown fat cells in many parts of the body. Their job is to regulate the amount of energy the body uses. Brown fat is a special fat that is fundamentally different from ordinary white fat both in composition and function. White fat is mainly an energy storage system where excess calories are deposited and stored for future use. Brown fat, on the other hand, is an energy-*using* material that is stimulated by the nervous system to burn up calories. Thus brown fat reduces the amount of white fat. Brown fat's primary task is to regulate and maintain our body temperature. As it uses energy much faster than other body cells, it is used to produce warmth in cold weather. When this warmth is not required it is dissipated. Brown fat also plays an important role in weight control by burning off excess calories.

White fat cells

White fat cells that are used to store fat in the body are called adipocytes. Even a lean person has between twenty and forty billion adipocytes. These are not simply inert storage vessels, they are active living cells. As they store fat, adipocytes swell, but they can only double in size, so there should be a limit to how much fat we can carry. Unfortunately for people who eat the wrong foods, Nature has thoughtfully provided us with a vast reserve of extremely small cells called preadipocytes of which we are completely unaware – until they mutate into adipocytes. After adipocytes have been used to store fat to their limit, preadipocytes are converted for use. Insulin, the hormone produced as a response to excessively high blood sugar levels, triggers this mutation. And once this happens you have the extra adipocytes for life: these fat cells can get smaller, but never fewer, a fact that has serious implications for successful weight-loss programmes.

The earlier in your life that you convert more preadipocytes into fat cells, the more difficult it will be to retain a normal weight. Not surprisingly, therefore, the most difficult form of obesity to correct is childhood onset obesity. People who were obese as children have a very hard time trying to lose weight and are much more likely to regain lost weight quickly.

The rhythm method of girth control

Using the controls outlined above, the healthy body can regulate very precisely the rate at which it uses fuel in conjunction with the amount ingested.

When you eat less than your appetite says you need, the first effect is that your appetite is not satisfied. This is abnormal and unnatural. If you continue, your appetite becomes blunted until eventually it no longer works - correctly. At the same time, if your energy intake is insufficient, you start to use up your energy stores and lose weight. But if your energy intake continues to be less than you need, the brown fat recognises that you are starving and reduces its activity. It conserves energy by slowing down the rate at which your body uses it. Other metabolic processes are also run more energy-efficiently. This is why the weight loss may be high at the start of a diet, but then becomes progressively less. And when you resume a 'normal' eating pattern, after the period of low-calorie dieting, your body takes the opportunity to store extra energy, in the form of fat, in case of more hard times to come.

This is the way to put weight on. A recent survey by European obesity experts showed that repeated dieting was a greater cause of obesity than lack of will power, inactivity or depression leading to overeating. Yo-yo dieting is probably the surest way to become overweight in later life.

The long-term effects of yo-yo dieting were studied in a cohort of 1,772 former elite male athletes and 651 healthy age-matched non-athletes who acted as controls. The athletes included 273 men engaged in power sports that forced them to yo-yo diet.

By 1985 the yo-yo dieting power athletes had put on much more weight than either the other athletes or the controls, and there were three times as many cases of clinical obesity in the yo-yo group as among the other athletes and twice as many as among the controls.

Similarly, a 1986 Dutch study showed that men who had experienced several weight changes within a short space of time put weight on. A year later this excess weight had disappeared in all subgroups except one: a group who had resorted to low-calorie dieting to lose their excess weight – they had put on even more weight!

This is why most people who diet get progressively fatter over the years. The process leads to ever more stringent diets, the brown fat is damaged, it atrophies and stops working.

Changing from one diet to another and alternating periods of dieting and normal eating weaken your weight-regulating mechanisms, making it necessary for you to undertake ever more stringent diets to achieve the same weight loss. This effect was demonstrated in a trial using subjects who had never dieted before. The first time they dieted they lost an average 1.5 kg (3 $\frac{1}{2}$ lb) a week, but they lost only 1 kg (2 $\frac{1}{2}$ lb) a week during their second diet.

Persistent low-calorie dieting can damage any of the control systems. Many people crave food all day. In them there may be damage to the 'switch-off' opiates, their appetite becomes defective and they are never satisfied. These are the people who cannot help nibbling between meals. There are others who get fat and yet eat very little (and have great difficulty in convincing their doctors of this). Here it is the activation of their brown fat that may be at fault. Eventually, both the opiate and the brown fat systems may become flawed.

Low-calorie dietary regimes invariably fail. More importantly, they damage your health, engender a feeling of disillusion and failure, lower morale and increase mental as well as physical stress.

Normalisation of controls

For the natural controls to work correctly they must be normalised. Appetite and hunger are natural and vital signals and both must be satisfied. Therefore no dietary regime should be harmful to the body. It should follow a pattern that is normal and natural.

Modern low-calorie diets, whether they are obviously faddy – relying on a very restricted range of nutrient-poor foods – or requiring a more subtle reduction of calorific intake, are abnormal. They all encourage hunger but do not satisfy it. Neither, usually, do they satisfy the appetite.

The most important prerequisite of any diet is to get the body's systems working normally again. If you are comparatively new to dieting, this should not be too big a problem. It may take a little longer, however, if you have been low-calorie dieting for many years. Nevertheless, it is never too late to begin eating properly.

4

The Cholesterol Myth

The tragedy of science is the slaying of a beautiful hypothesis by an ugly fact.
T. H. HUXLEY

The BMA and the Government recommend that the British people should drink eighty per cent more milk, eat fifty-five per cent more eggs, forty per cent more butter and thirty per cent more meat.

On the basis of research in the 1920s and 1930s by Sir John Boyd Orr and others, that was the advice given to the British people in 1938. The Government introduced free school milk – full cream, that is – and later we 'went to work on an egg'. As a consequence, child deaths from diphtheria, measles, scarlet fever and whooping cough fell dramatically, well before the introduction of antibiotics and widespread immunisation. Rickets, called 'the English Disease' because it was so widespread, and other deficiency diseases were relegated to the past. Other factors helped, but most important of all was the better nutrition that gave children a higher resistance. The recommendations above shaped our diet for nearly fifty years and helped to give us a mean life expectancy that is now among the highest in the world. Sixty years in 1930, our mean life expectancy had climbed to seventy by 1960 and to seventy-five by 1990.

Now we are told meat and dairy products are shortening our lives, killing us with coronary heart disease. Why the sudden change? To discover that, we need to know something of the history of coronary heart disease and how the strategy to combat it evolved.

Coronary heart disease

There are many diseases that affect the heart but the one that the 'healthy eating' strategies seek to prevent is Coronary Heart Disease (CHD), more correctly called ischaemic heart disease (IHD). CHD is a condition where the coronary arteries that supply blood to nourish the heart muscle are narrowed by a build-up of material on their walls (an atheroma) to such an extent that they become blocked. This cuts off the blood supply to part of the heart muscle, causing a heart attack. The narrowing also encourages the clotting of blood and, in consequence, it is possible for a clot to cause a heart attack long before the atheroma is large enough to do so. The material generally blamed for the build-up is cholesterol and the 'healthy eating' advice given to the public to reduce the incidence of CHD is aimed simply at reducing the levels of cholesterol in the blood.

Cholesterol

Because of the propaganda, you can be forgiven for thinking that cholesterol is a harmful alien substance that should be avoided at all costs. In fact, nothing could be further from the truth. Cholesterol is an essential component in the body. It is found in all the cells of the body, particularly in the brain and nerve cells. Body cells are continually dying and new ones being made. Cholesterol is a major building block from which cell walls are made. Cholesterol is also used to make a number of other important substances: hormones (including the sex hormones), bile acids and, in conjunction with sunlight on the skin, vitamin D_3. The body uses large quantities of cholesterol every day and the substance is so important that, with the exception of brain cells, every body cell has the ability to make it.

Cholesterol may be ingested in animal products, but less than twenty per cent of your body's cholesterol needs will be supplied in this way. Your body then makes up the difference. If you eat less cholesterol, your body merely compensates by making more. Although the media and food companies still warn against cholesterol in diet, it has been repeatedly demonstrated that the level of cholesterol in your blood is very little affected by the amount of cholesterol you eat.

Cholesterol and CHD

For reasons still unknown, in the 1920s coronary heart disease suddenly became widespread in the industrialised world. By the 1940s it was becoming the major cause of premature death. And nobody knew why.

In 1950 an American doctor, John Gofman, hypothesised that blood cholesterol was to blame. His theory was supported in 1951 when pathologists were sent to Korea to learn about war wounds by dissecting the bodies of dead soldiers. To their surprise they discovered unexpected evidence of CHD: unexpected for they knew that death from heart disease was extremely rare under middle age and these men averaged only twenty-two years of age. So the pathologists performed detailed dissections on the hearts of the next 300 corpses. In thirty-five per cent they found deposits of fibrous, fatty material sticking to the artery walls. A further forty-one per cent had fully formed lesions, and in three per cent of the soldiers these lesions were sufficiently large to block at least one coronary artery. Thus, over three-quarters of all the men examined showed evidence of serious coronary heart disease – and they were barely out of their teens.

Doctors now had a problem. As there are no symptoms with the partial blockage of the coronary arteries, how could they tell, without resorting to surgery, who was in danger? They had to find out how those with the disease differed from those free of it.

To cut a long story short, they found cholesterol in the material that builds up on artery walls and causes them to become blocked; people who died of heart disease often had high levels of cholesterol in their blood; and those who suffered the rare hereditary disease, *familial hyper-cholesterolaemia* (hereditary high blood cholesterol), also suffered a higher incidence of CHD. And so, not unnaturally perhaps, cholesterol and heart disease became linked.

But there are a number of significant points that the cholesterol theory overlooks. For example, there is a marked difference between the build-up found in those with familial hyper-cholesterolaemia and those with coronary heart disease: hyper-cholesterolaemia causes large deposits at the mouths of the coronary arteries, often leaving the arteries themselves unblocked, and so does not reproduce the type of obstruction found in coronary heart disease. It has also long been known that simple events, such as putting a cuff around the arm prior to taking a blood sample, or fear of the needle, can result in raised cholesterol values.

Cholesterol testing

One of the effects of the 'fight or flight' reflex is rapidly to raise blood cholesterol. Any form of physical or mental stress has this effect. So if you run to your doctor's, your cholesterol level will be higher than if you walked; if you are anxious, or your doctor looks worried, it will be higher. If your blood cholesterol were tested hourly throughout a day, or daily over a month, it would not be unusual to find a wide variation in values.

Blood cholesterol levels also rise naturally as you get older so that while a reading of 9 mmol/l is high at the age of twenty, it is perfectly normal if you are fifty.

The accuracy of cholesterol measurements is not very high – less than eighty per cent – even when conducted in a laboratory. A survey showed that on the same sample, laboratories could differ by as much as 1.2 mmol/l. When cholesterol levels are tested with a doctor's desktop machine the accuracy will inevitably be lower.

In fact, so many variables affect cholesterol levels that a one-off test is a waste of time, and an unnecessary worry for the patient that can do more harm than good. Bear that in mind if you are subjected to a cholesterol test.

Dietary intervention

That diet might play a part in causing CHD was hypothesised by another American doctor, Ancel Keys, in 1953. In his 'Seven Countries Study', Keys compared the death rates from CHD and the amounts of fats eaten in the selected countries to demonstrate that heart disease mortality was higher in those where more fat was consumed. (It seems that Keys ignored the substantial available data from other countries which did not support his hypothesis.) And so the 'diet/heart' hypothesis was born. But how do we know it is correct? In medicine, the usual way to prove a theory involves studying two groups of people, as identical for sex, age, and lifestyle as possible. One group, called the *control group*, carries on as normal while the other, called the *intervention group*, tries the new diet, drug or whatever. After a suitable time, the two groups are compared and differences noted.

Keys' fat-diet/heart disease hypothesis was persuasive so, to test it, several large-scale, long-term human intervention studies were set up in many parts of the world. These involved hundreds of thousands of subjects and hundreds of doctors and scientists and cost billions of dollars in an attempt to prove that a fatty diet caused heart disease.

The Framingham Heart Study

The most influential and respected investigation of the causes of heart disease is the Framingham Heart Study. This study was set up in the town of Framingham, Massachusetts, by Harvard University Medical School in 1948 and is still going on today. It was this study that produced the dietary 'risk factors' with which we all are so familiar today. The Framingham researchers thought that they knew exactly why some people had more cholesterol than others – they ate more in their diet. To prove the link, they measured cholesterol intake and compared it with blood cholesterol. As the table below shows, although subjects consumed wide-ranging amounts of cholesterol, there was little or no difference in the levels of cholesterol in their blood and, thus, no relationship between the amount of cholesterol eaten and levels of blood cholesterol was found.

Next, the scientists studied intakes of saturated fats but again they could find no correlation. Nor could any be found when they studied total calorie intake. They then considered the possibility that something was masking the effects of diet, but no other factor made the slightest difference.

Cholesterol intake – The Framingham Heart Study

	Cholesterol intake mg/day	Blood cholesterol in those below median intake	above median intake
		mmol/l	
Men	704 ± 220.9	6.16	6.16
Women	492 ± 170.0	6.37	6.26

After twenty-two years' research, the researchers concluded: 'There is, in short, no suggestion of any relation between diet and the subsequent development of CHD in the study group.'

Subsequent research findings

On Christmas Eve, 1997, after a further twenty-seven years, the *Journal of the American Medical Association* (JAMA) carried a follow-up report that showed that dietary saturated fat reduced strokes. As these tend to affect older men than CHD, they wondered if a fatty diet was causing those in the trial to die of CHD before they had a stroke. But the researchers discount this, saying:

> This hypothesis, however, depends on the presence of a strong direct association of fat intake with coronary heart disease. Since we found no such association, competing mortality from coronary heart disease is very unlikely to explain our results.

In other words, after forty-nine years of research, scientists are unable to find a relation between a fatty diet and heart disease. A review of twenty-six studies published in 1992 concluded: Lowering serum cholesterol concentrations does not reduce mortality and is unlikely to prevent coronary heart disease.

One study that seemed to support the 'healthy' recommendations was a Finnish trial published in 1975. In the five years that the trial ran, cholesterol levels were lowered significantly. But in December 1991 the results of a ten-year follow-up to that trial found that those people who continued to follow the carefully controlled, cholesterol-lowering diet were *twice* as likely to die of heart disease as those who didn't.

Experience in other countries

Keys based his fat-causes-heart-disease hypothesis on a comparison between countries. We in Britain are described as 'the sick man of Europe' in comparison to other countries. So let's examine the facts.

1. In Japan, intakes of animal fat have more than doubled since the end of the Second World War. Over the same period their incidence of coronary heart disease has fallen consistently.

2. In Israel too an increased consumption of saturated fats was followed by a fall in coronary deaths.

3. The dietary changes in Sweden parallel those in the USA, yet heart disease mortality in Sweden was rising while American rates were falling.

4. There is also a threefold variation in rates of heart disease between France and Finland even though fat intake in those two countries is very similar.

5. Among south Asians in Britain there is an unusually high incidence of heart disease, yet living on largely vegetarian diets, they have low levels of blood cholesterol and eat diets that are low in saturated fat.

6. Indians in South Africa have probably the highest rates of coronary disease in the world, for no apparent reason that fits the current dietary hypotheses.

7. Until recently, Indians in India had a very low incidence of heart disease while using ghee (clarified butter), coconut oil and mustard seed oil, all of which are highly saturated. The epidemic of heart disease in India began only after these were replaced with peanut, safflower, sunflower, sesame and soybean oils, all of which are high in polyunsaturated oils.

8. Lastly, the World Health Organisation is apparently in ignorance of epidemiological data that do not support its recommendation to reduce dietary saturated fat. While it suggests that coronary heart disease is responsible for most deaths in Caribbean countries, fat intake there is remarkably low.

Polyunsaturated fats

The arguments for the polyunsaturated fat hypothesis are no more convincing than those for the cholesterol theory. The claim is that unsaturated fats have a protective or preventative effect on CHD. But in Israel, when consumption of polyunsaturated fats was about twice that of most Western countries, there was a very high incidence of CHD. Those given high polyunsaturated diets in a trial in New South Wales fared significantly worse than those on a free diet. And this is the finding in most trials that have increased the ratio of polyunsaturated fats.

From as early as 1971, an excess of cancer deaths has been reported in trials using diets that were high in polyunsaturated fats. Polyunsaturated fats are also blamed for a doubling in the incidence of gallstones in the general public.

One of the pioneers of the polyunsaturated-fat-prevents-CHD hypothesis was the American cardiologist E. H. Ahrens Jr. After twenty-five years of further research, however, he concluded that it was 'irresponsible' to

continue to press the polyunsaturated fat recommendations on the general public.

Another of the original proponents of the low-fat, low-
cholesterol hypothesis, and a member of the Norwegian
Council for Diseases of the Heart and Arteries, Professor
Jens Dedichen of Oslo, also changed his mind – and
received a very hostile reaction from his colleagues. In the
1950s Norway launched a cholesterol-lowering regimen in
which soy margarine, high in polyunsaturated fatty acids,
replaced butter, and soy oil was used extensively. During
the subsequent twenty years the increase in the use of
soy-based products was accompanied by a steep and
continuing rise in deaths from coronary thrombosis.

Margarine – a natural food?

The polyunsaturated fats used to make margarine are
generally obtained from vegetable sources such as
sunflower seed, cottonseed, and soy bean. As such they
might be thought of as natural foods. Usually, however,
they are sold in the form of highly processed margarines,
spreads and oils and, as such, they are anything but
natural.

In 1989, the petroleum-based solvent, benzene, which is
known to cause cancer, was found in Perrier mineral
water at a mean concentration of fourteen parts per
billion. This was enough to cause Perrier to be removed
from supermarket shelves. The first process in the
manufacture of margarine is the extraction of the oils
from the seeds, and this is usually done using similar
petroleum-based solvents. Although these are then boiled
off, this stage of the process still leaves about ten parts per
million of the solvents in the product. That is 700 times
as much as fourteen parts per billion.

The oils then go through more than ten other processes
– degumming, bleaching, hydrogenation, neutralization,

fractionation, deodorisation, emulsification, interesterification – that include heat treatment at 140° to 160° C with a solution of caustic soda; the use of nickel, a metal that is known to cause cancer, as a catalyst, with up to fifty parts per million of the nickel left in the product; the addition of antioxidants such as butylated hydroxyanisol (E320). These antioxidants are again usually petroleum based and are widely believed to cause cancer. The hydrogenation process that solidifies the oils so that they are spreadable produces *trans*-fatty acids that rarely occur in nature.

The heat treatment alone is enough to render these margarines nutritionally inadequate. When the massive chemical treatment and unnatural fats are added, the end product can hardly be called either natural or healthy.

Recent US studies showed that heart disease worsened in those who switched from butter to polyunsaturate-rich margarine. Research published in March 1993 confirmed this. In a study that involved 85,000 nurses, women who ate just four teaspoons of polyunsaturated margarine a day had a sixty-six per cent *increased* risk of CHD compared to those who ate none – and CHD is the one disease eating this sort of margarine was supposed to reduce!

INGREDIENTS THAT MAY BE PRESENT IN BUTTER AND MARGARINE:

Butter
  milk fat (cream)
  a little salt

Margarine
  edible oils
  edible fats
  salt or potassium chloride
  ascorbyl palmitate
  butylated hydroxyanisole

phospholipids
tert-butylhydroquinone
mono- and di-glycerides of fat-forming fatty acids
disodium guanylate
diacetyltartaric and fatty acid esters of glycerol
Propyl octyl or dodecyl gallate (or mixtures thereof)
tocopherols
propylene glycol mono- and di-esters
sucrose esters of fatty acids
curcumin
annatto extracts
tartaric acid
35trimethylhexanal
ß-apo-carotenoic acid methyl or ethyl ester
skim milk powder
xanthophylls
canthaxanthin
vitamins A and D.

Dietary fat patterns

The total amount of fats in our diet today, according to the MAFF National Food Survey, is almost the same as it was at the beginning of this century. What has changed, to some extent, is the types of fats eaten. At the turn of the century we ate mainly animal fats that are largely saturated and monounsaturated. Now we are tending to eat more polyunsaturated fats – it's what we are advised to do. In 1991, two studies, from USA and Canada, found that linoleic acid, the major polyunsaturated fatty acid found in vegetable oils, increased the risk of breast tumours.

Body cell walls are made of cholesterol. We contain very little polyunsaturated fat. Cell walls have to allow the various nutrients that body cells need from the blood, but stop harmful pathogens. They must be stable. An intake of large quantities of polyunsaturated fatty acids changes the constituency of cholesterol and body fat. Cell walls become softer and more unstable. As Professor Raymond Kearney of Sydney University put it in 1987: 'Vegetable oils (e.g. corn oil and sunflower oil) which are rich in linoleic acid are potent promoters of tumour growth.'

Carcinogens – background radiation, ultraviolet radiation from the sun, particles in the air we breathe and the food we eat – continually attack us all. Normally, the immune system deals with any small focus of cancer cells so formed and that is the end of it. But linoleic acid suppresses the immune system. Indeed it is so good at this that in the 1970s sunflower oil was given to kidney transplant patients to prevent kidneys being rejected – until an excess of cancer deaths was reported. With a high intake of margarine, therefore, a tumour may grow too rapidly for the weakened immune system to cope, thus increasing our risk of a cancer.

Fats and melanoma

Since 1974, the increase of polyunsaturated fats has been blamed for the alarming increase in malignant melanoma (skin cancer) in Australia. We are all told that the sun causes it. Are Australians going out in the sun any more now than they were fifty years ago? They are certainly eating more polyunsaturated oils: even milk has its cream removed and replaced with vegetable oil. Victims of the disease have been found to have polyunsaturated oils in their skin cells. Polyunsaturated oils are oxidised readily by ultraviolet radiation from the sun and form harmful 'free radicals'. These are known to damage the cell's DNA and this can lead to the deregulation we call cancer. Saturated fats are stable. They do not oxidise and form free radicals.

Malignant melanoma is also said to be increasing in this country. Does the sun cause this? In Britain the number of sufferers is so small as to be relatively insignificant. Even so, it is not likely that the sun is to blame since all the significant increase is among those aged over seventy-five. People in this age group tend to get very little sun.

Melanoma occurs ten times as often in Orkney and Shetland as it does on Mediterranean islands. It also occurs more frequently on areas that are *not* exposed to the sun. In Scotland, for example, there are five times as many melanomas on the feet as on the hands; and in Japan, forty per cent of pedal melanomas are on the soles of the feet.

. . . and breast cancer

A study of 61,471 women aged forty to seventy-six, conducted in Sweden, looked into different fats in relation to breast cancer. The results were published in January 1998. This study found an inverse association with monounsaturated fat and a positive association with polyunsaturated fat. In other words, monounsaturated fats protected against breast cancer and polyunsaturated fats increased the risk. Saturated fats were neutral.

Linoleic acid and CHD

Flora margarine, the brand leader, is thirty-nine per cent linoleic acid; Vitalite and other 'own brand' polyunsaturated margarines are similar. Of cooking oils, sunflower oil is fifty per cent and safflower oil seventy-two per cent linoleic acid. Butter, on the other hand, has only a mere two per cent and lard is just nine per cent linoleic acid. Linoleic acid is one of the essential fatty acids. We must eat some to live, but we do not need much. That found in animal fats is quite sufficient.

Because of the heart disease risk, in 1994 the manufacturers of Flora changed its formula to cut out the trans fats and other manufacturers have since followed. But that still leaves the linoleic acid.

The anti-cancer fat

Linoleic acid is one of the essential fatty acids that our bodies need but cannot synthesise. We must eat some to survive. Fortunately there is one form of linoleic acid that is beneficial. Conjugated linoleic acid (CLA) differs from the normal form of linoleic acid only in the position of two of the bonds that join its atoms. But this small difference has been shown to give it powerful anti-cancer properties.

Conjugated linoleic acid has one other difference from the usual form: it is not found in vegetables but in the fat of ruminant animals. The best sources are dairy products and the fat on red meat, principally beef. It is another good reason not to give up eating red meat or to cut off the fat.

Scientists at the University of Wisconsin also believe that CLA has a slimming action. They put the dramatic increase in obesity in the USA down to Americans not eating beef fat.

Monounsaturated fats

Several populations in the world, Eskimos and those in the Mediterranean countries for example, eat high-fat diets yet have very low incidences of heart disease. This realisation has led to research scientists switching their attention to monounsaturated fats found in fish oils and olive oil.

Although the supposed virtues of monounsaturated fats are being talked of in the press as possible saviours of Western man, the monounsaturated theory is not new. It was first demonstrated over thirty years ago that giving people more unsaturated fats could lower blood cholesterol. However, surveys of countries with different tastes in fats and oils have failed to show that this protects against heart disease. For example, Norwegians, who eat a lot of saturated fats, have lower rates of the disease than New Zealanders who eat a similar amount. But if, as has been suggested, the Norwegians are protected by the monounsaturated oils in the fish that they eat, then why is it that in Aberdeen, where a lot of fish is also consumed, the heart disease rate is double that of Oslo? Proponents forget that many other people, such as the Maasai tribes of Africa, who eat neither fish nor olive oil, have a low incidence of heart disease too.

There is no evidence that either mono- or polyunsaturated oils are of benefit to those who have already suffered a heart attack. As long ago as 1965 survival rates were studied in patients eating different oils. Splitting patients into three groups, who were given polyunsaturated corn oil, monounsaturated olive oil and saturated animal fats respectively, it was found that only the corn oil lowered blood cholesterol levels. At first sight, therefore, it seemed that men in the polyunsaturated group had the best chance of survival. However, at the end of the two-year trial only fifty-two per cent of the polyunsaturated corn oil group were still alive and free of a fresh heart attack. Those on the monounsaturated olive oil fared little better: fifty-seven per cent survived and had no further attack. Those eating the saturated animal fats, however, fared much better with seventy-five per cent surviving and without a further attack.

Low blood cholesterol and cancer

So far advertisers and news media have concentrated on the supposed danger of high levels of blood cholesterol. The dangers of low blood cholesterol levels have largely been ignored.

Countries with diets high in saturated fats also tend to have high levels of colon cancer. In 1974 a review of the Framingham data and those from Keys' 'Seven Countries Study' was carried out. It was expected to show that the cancer could also be blamed on high blood cholesterol. However, the baffled researchers found the opposite: those with the cancer had cholesterol levels that were *lower* than average.

Reports of more than twenty studies into the relation between blood cholesterol and cancer have been published since 1972. Most have reported an association between low blood cholesterol and cancer. The authors of the Renfrew and Paisley Study conclude: 'It may be a mistake to assume that dietary advice given to the general population to reduce the intake of saturated fat will necessarily reduce overall mortality.'

More cholesterol means fewer strokes

A very large study in Japan, covering two decades, recently concluded that low levels of blood cholesterol also increase the incidence of stroke. Over the past few decades, Japan has experienced a rapid change in its living and eating patterns. The Japanese are eating more total fat, saturated fatty acids and cholesterol, animal fats and protein, and less rice and vegetables. This has provided a unique opportunity for a large-scale natural experiment into the effects of those changes.

Investigators have shown that this change to Western and urban eating patterns, departing as it does from centuries old traditions, has been accompanied by a general lowering of blood pressure and a large decline in the incidence of stroke deaths and cerebral haemorrhage between the 1960s and the 1980s. They attribute this decline to an increase in blood cholesterol levels over the period. Supporting their findings were the results of a follow-up of 350,000 men screened for the MRFIT in the United States which showed that the risk of death from cerebral haemorrhage in middle-aged men was six times greater if they had low blood cholesterol levels.

Low cholesterol and childhood mortality

In 1991 the US national cholesterol education programme recommended that children over two years old should adopt a low-fat, low-cholesterol diet to prevent CHD in later life. A table showing a good correlation between fat and cholesterol intakes and blood cholesterol in seven- to nine-year-old boys from six countries supported this advice. What it did not show, however, was the strong correlation between blood cholesterol and childhood deaths in those countries (see table below). As is clearly demonstrated, the death rate rises dramatically as blood cholesterol levels fall. So for children, too, low blood cholesterol is unhealthy.

BLOOD CHOLESTEROL AND MORTALITY IN UNDER-FIVES IN SIX COUNTRIES

	Blood cholesterol deaths	Childhood deaths
Finland	4.9	7
Netherlands	4.5	9
USA	4.3	12
Italy	4.1	12
Philippines	3.8	72
Ghana	3.3	145

. . . and at the other end of life

Two studies which considered total blood cholesterol levels and mortality in the elderly were published in the *Lancet* almost simultaneously in 1997. In the first, scientists working at the Leiden University Medical Centre found that 'each 1 mmol/l increase in total cholesterol corresponded to a 15% decrease in mortality'. Similarly, doctors at Reykjavik Hospital and Heart Disease Preventive Clinic in Iceland noted that the major epidemiological studies had not included the elderly. They too studied total mortality and blood cholesterol in the over-eighties and showed that the mortality rate for men with blood cholesterol levels over 6.5 was less than half that of those whose cholesterol level was around 5.2.

Low cholesterol and Alzheimer's Disease

Approximately half of the brain is made up of fats. Dr F. M. Corrigan and colleagues, writing in 1991 about the relief of Alzheimer's Disease, ask that 'strategies for increasing the delivery of cholesterol to the brain should be identified'. In the fight against Alzheimer's disease, they recommend increasing fat intake.

Has anyone gained?

So far we have been looking at cholesterol lowering in terms of numbers of deaths, but the trials have shown impressive results in the reduction of non-fatal heart attacks and a consequent improvement in the quality of life. In the case of drugs, the reduction was in the order of twenty-three per cent. Many see this as proof that lowering cholesterol in the total population, by whatever means, is worth fighting for.

But those trials were conducted on men rather than women. They were also conducted on those who had hypercholesterolaemia or, at least, very high blood cholesterol levels – not on people with normal levels. They ignore the now well-established, non-linear relation between blood cholesterol and heart disease which indicates that lowering blood cholesterol in the general population is not economically worthwhile. The widespread agreement that the focus of the campaign should be a change in diet and lifestyle for all also overlooks the complete lack of evidence that such a course would have any significant beneficial effect. It even overlooks the fact that the trials involving cholesterol lowering by dietary means did not show any significant reductions in blood cholesterol.

In 1992 a report of nineteen major studies published over the past twenty years suggested that public policy for reducing blood cholesterol should be reviewed. The table below plots the relative mortality risk from all causes associated with levels of blood cholesterol in men and women. In the case of women, you can see clearly that risk rises as blood cholesterol falls. The report's author, Dr Hulley, states: 'We are coming to realise that the resulting cardiovascular research, which represents the great majority of the effort so far, may not apply to women.'

With men, the situation is more complicated, as the curve is U-shaped. However, it is still noticeable that the risk with low cholesterol is similar to the risk with high cholesterol. Dr Hulley concludes:

> The findings call into question policies built over several decades on evidence that focused only on CHD as an outcome . . . it may be time to review national policies aimed at shifting the entire population distribution of blood cholesterol to the left.

TOTAL MORTALITY AND BLOOD CHOLESTEROL

Blood cholesterol (mmol/l)	Health hazard ratio	
	men	women
<4.16	1.17	1.10
4.16–5.2	1.00	1.00
5.2–6.2	1.02	0.96
>6.2	1.16	0.97

Another analysis based on a number of American studies estimated that on a lifelong programme of cholesterol reduction by diet, the gain in life expectancy for those at very high risk (that is the one in 500 with hypercholesterolaemia) would be between eighteen days and twelve months, and for those at low risk (that is the other 499) between three days and three months. That is not very much with which to tempt people to endure a lifetime of unpalatable diets. And these figures assumed that cholesterol lowering was both effective and safe; they didn't take into account the increased risk of other debilitating and fatal diseases. Once these are added to the equation, it becomes quite evident that the current campaign is certain to do more harm than good. A study of Maoris in New Zealand showed that those with the *lowest* levels of blood cholesterol had the *highest* mortality, findings also borne out by the Framingham Study.

Summary

- A number of very large-scale, long-term human intervention studies show that lowering blood cholesterol is possible but that it has no beneficial effect on coronary heart disease in the general population.

- Other studies show that a low blood cholesterol level, or the methods used to attain it, are increasing the incidence of other serious killer diseases.

- Thirty years ago it was said that 'current medical thinking . . . is that while cholesterol may be involved in some way with arteriosclerosis and heart disease, it is no longer held to be the main factor'. And 'A recent survey of cholesterol findings in geriatric cases involving arteriosclerosis showed a significant number of patients to have normal or low cholesterol.' Those remarks have been confirmed by all the major studies published to date.

- Forty years after the Framingham Heart Study began, its researchers looked at total mortality and cholesterol. The evidence was that for those with low cholesterol levels, deaths from non-cardiac causes offset any reduced incidence of heart disease. There was 'no increased overall mortality with either high or low serum cholesterol levels' among men over forty-seven years of age. There was no relationship with women older than forty-seven or younger than forty. The researchers also concluded that people whose cholesterol levels are falling may be at *increased* risk.

- And ten years later the Framingham researchers say: 'Intakes of fat and type of fat were not related to the incidence of the combined outcome of all cardiovascular diseases or to total or cardiovascular mortality.'

- Thus we now have fifty years of studies all demonstrating that *animal fat is harmless*.

So where does this leave coronary heart disease?

Is coronary heart disease really the major killer it's made out to be? It is true that a large percentage of deaths in Britain are attributed to CHD. The question is: is this a cause for concern? As you can see in the table below, CHD deaths have increased in people over seventy-five years of age. But does this illustrate a problem?

It is a fallacy to believe that if these people had modified their diet or lifestyle, they would still be alive. Despite what the health industry tells us, we are not an immortal species and cannot expect to live for ever. I suggest that these figures merely show that people tended to live longer in 1995 than in 1975. This is true of both sexes and that, surely, is a good thing.

CHD MORTALITY IN UK OVER AGE 70 BY SEX AND AGE

Ages	70–74	75–79	80–84	Over 85
Men				
1975	16297	12561	8666	6270
1995	13379	12975	12223	10254
Women				
1975	10598	12868	12589	14617
1995	7695	9915	13717	21263

ICD 410-414

Premature death from CHD is a legitimate cause for concern. If dietary change can reduce premature deaths it is arguably to their advantage that people be urged to change their ways. However, the table below illustrates clearly that CHD deaths have fallen considerably in all under-seventy age groups and both sexes over the past two decades. Some say that this is evidence that 'healthy eating' is working.

CHD MORTALITY IN **UK** UNDER AGE **70** BY SEX AND AGE

Ages	40–44	45–49	50–54	55–59	60–64	65–69
Men						
1975	1290	2914	5783	7214	11678	15448
1995	643	1473	2261	3766	6170	9591
Women						
1975	202	473	1072	1902	3950	7104
1995	124	262	480	979	2028	4188

ICD 410-414

Do not be misled. This reduction cannot be the result of the 'healthy diet' recommendations – they only began with the COMA report of 1984, but *premature* CHD deaths had started to decline nearly twenty years before in 1965, as is graphically illustrated in the table above.

This was a time when people were brought up or spent the greater part of their lives with the recommendations with which this chapter began. They had free full-cream milk at school, ate bread and dripping and fried breakfasts. During the period after World War II when deaths from CHD peaked and started to fall, rationing had ended and a diet that was relatively high in fat was the norm.

CORONARY DEATHS, MEN AGED 40–44
(ICD 410-414)

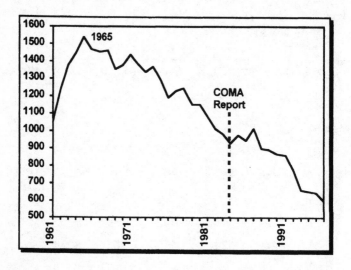

Not that this will come as any surprise to the Medical Research Council. In its report on the Caerphilly Study published in 1993, the MRC's Epidemiology Unit at Cardiff showed that men who drank more than a pint of full-cream milk a day had only one-tenth the incidence of heart disease of those who drank none. They also demonstrated that those who ate a high-energy diet lived longer than those who cut dietary fats. Their findings indicate that far from being a killer, the diet we are told to avoid by the nutritionists may actually protect us against heart disease!

These findings confirmed a Japanese study of 1992. Japan has low levels of death from coronary heart disease, but Okinawa has the lowest of all. While blood cholesterol levels are generally low in Japan, Okinawa's levels are much higher, similar to those in Scotland. In 1994 a paper examined the relationship of nutritional status to further life expectancy and health in the Japanese elderly based on three epidemiological studies. It found that Japanese who lived to the age of one hundred were those who got their protein from meat rather than from rice and pulses. The centenarians also had higher intakes of animal foods such as eggs, milk, meat and fish. Significantly, their carbohydrate intake was lower than that of their fellow countrymen who died younger.

The Mediterranean diet

The 'Mediterranean' diet is healthier than ours, we are told. We should eat what the French, Italians and Spanish eat. That could be right, but not for the reasons usually given.

The Mediterranean diet is what the health fanatics advocate because, they say, it is low in fat. This is nonsense! Obviously, they have never been there. Northern Italians love butter, bowls of pork dripping are sold in Spanish markets and the Spanish spread it thickly on their toast for breakfast. Goose fat is used to make *cassoulet* in the south of France, and throughout the Mediterranean sausages, salamis and pâtés all contain up to fifty per cent fat.

The Mediterranean diet may be healthier than the British but, contrary to popular belief, it is very far from being a low-fat diet!

However, there are a number of major differences between the Mediterranean countries and Britain that may have a significant effect on health. Not only is the food eaten by the average working family in southern Europe very different from that eaten by a typical family in Britain, more importantly, it differs in the way it is bought, presented and eaten. A brief list of the principal differences is tabled below.

Mediterranean eating pattern	British eating pattern
• The average Mediterranean diet comprises natural, unprocessed meat, vegetables and fruit that are usually bought fresh daily.	• The average British diet is composed of packaged, highly processed foods with chemical additives.
• Meat plays an important part in the diet.	• In Britain we are told to eat less meat.
• Fats eaten are butter, olive oil and unprocessed animal fats.	• Fats eaten are highly processed margarines, low-fat fat substitutes, and vegetable oils.
• Meals are taken slowly, without hurrying. Lunch usually takes up to two hours, and is followed by a siesta.	• Food is rushed. Lunches are eaten on the run or combined with work. Often, they are junk-food snacks.
• Over sixty per cent of energy intake occurs before 2 p.m.	• The largest meal is eaten in the evening.
• Wine (believed to be protective against heart disease) is drunk during meals as part of the meal.	• Beer, wines and spirits are drunk in the evening after the evening meal.

Conclusions

More resources, time and money have been spent over the last fifty years on coronary heart disease than any other disease in medical history and all it has proved is that doctors don't know as much as they thought they did. If half a century of serious research has failed to find a causal link between a fatty diet and heart disease, it can only be because there is no link.

To make intelligent decisions you must be given advice that is based on proven facts rather than unfounded assumptions. And the facts at present seem to be that *milk, cream, butter, meat and fresh fruit and vegetables are the healthy foods* whilst high-in-polyunsaturates spreads and oils, bran flakes and packaged foods are not.

Seventy years after it began we still do not know what caused the dramatic rise in coronary heart disease deaths of the 1920s or why coronary mortality is now falling. But one thing that the last fifty years of research has demonstrated is that cholesterol has had very little to do with it.

The research has also demonstrated no evidence of a need to endure an unpalatable, fatless, bran-laden diet. Apart from being less pleasurable to eat, it is now clear that 'healthy eating' is not so healthy after all.

In 1979 the late Professor Sir John McMichael performed an inquest on the diet/heart hypothesis. Pointing out that 'All published efforts to help by drug or dietary reduction of blood cholesterol have uniformly and convincingly failed,' he concluded:

> We need a fresh approach to the problem at scientific level and should avoid further public speculation and confusion by repeated propaganda through the media until we have clarified our own professional minds and shaken off what

most critical doctors are likely to regard as an untenable
hypothesis of causation.

It is a pity that no one seems to have taken any notice of
Professor McMichael.

Fat has over twice the energy value of either
carbohydrates or proteins, and other essential nutrients:
lipids used in the brain and central nervous system
without which we become irritable and aggressive; sterols,
precursors of the bile acids and a number of hormones
(including the sex hormones); and the fat-soluble vitamins
A, D, E and K. The late Dr John Yudkin, when Professor of
Nutrition and Dietetics at London University, called fat
'the most valuable food known to man'. It is both stupid
and wasteful to throw it away.

5
Is Exercise Necessary?

You may enjoy exercise; it may be helpful socially; it may make you look and feel better. But all the rest is myth.
DR HENRY SOLOMON, CARDIOLOGIST,
CORNELL UNIVERSITY MEDICAL COLLEGE

How much exercise is natural?

If you watch animals in the wild you will see that on the whole, they take as little exercise as possible. The lion, for example, spends most of his day lying down or asleep, yet he doesn't get fat. It is his wife, the lioness, who is the hunter. But she hunts only once every two or three days and even then expends as little energy as possible doing it. Similarly, grazing animals have a slow and steady lifestyle, moving quickly only when threatened by a predator. The same is true of modern hunter-gatherer human tribes. In the wild, nature protects the heart from stress.

The combination of exercise and thinness is a well-established stereotype. The overweight are frequently criticised for not taking up the more strenuous physical activities enjoyed by slimmer people. Drs Andrew Prentice and Susan Jebb have pointed out that between 1980 and 1991 calorie intake in Britain fell by some 20 per cent, while the number of people who were overweight doubled. As we seem to be heeding the current dietary advice to eat less, but are nevertheless getting fatter,

Prentice and Jebb conclude that the overweight must be lazy.

Most modern diets advocate the twin strategies of taking in less energy (calorie-counting) while at the same time using more (exercising). And so slimmers are urged to take up some form of physical activity to burn up the calories. Not only will this help them to lose weight, they are told, it will make them fitter and healthier. Nonsense!

'Fitness' is a billion-pound industry which promotes books, exercise machinery, weights, footwear, clothing, and expensive gyms and clubs. If someone tells you that you need to exercise, you would be wise to question whether there is any commercial bias behind their advice.

Sport and exercise of the right kind can be rewarding both as a social outlet and in making you feel good, it may boost your self-esteem if you treat it as a form of group therapy, and it helps to keep muscles in trim and give your body a better shape. As such it has an important role to play, particularly as leisure time for most of us is increasing. This chapter is not anti-exercise. But it is against exercise as a means of achieving permanent weight loss – because it simply doesn't work.

A great deal of research has been carried out in the hope of demonstrating that exercise reduces weight in the obese and prevents weight gain. It has been consistently unsuccessful and very few studies have tried to discover why. Here are the results of some of them:

1. In 1976 Dr Per Björntorp and colleagues at the University of Gothenburg, Sweden, studied normal and overweight subjects on a six-month course of physical training. Although those at normal weight did lose weight on this programme, the overweight ones didn't.

2. Two years later Dr Martin Krotkiewski and colleagues conducted a similar study. They found that while mildly obese patients did tend to lose weight, severely obese

patients actually put on weight. These findings were not confined to Scandinavia.

3. In 1989 Drs J.-F. Yale, L. A. Leiter and E. B. Marliss, at McGill University, Montreal, and the University of Toronto, also found that exercise was fattening. Measuring blood insulin levels, they discovered that these remained much higher in obese patients for more than an hour after exercising. This means that their bodies were taking glucose out of the blood and storing it as glycogen and fat.

Studies published in the early 1990s found no causal relationship between low physical activity and obesity in either children or the elderly.

Exercise and energy stores

It may be possible to lose a small amount of weight by exercising. But this kind of weight loss is costly, short term, potentially dangerous and self-defeating. If, when you exercise, you burn up less energy than the amount of easily accessible glycogen stored in the liver and muscles, you won't use up any of your body fat – and therefore won't lose any weight. If you use more energy than is immediately available, any weight lost is at a cost of stress on your body.

The formula is another form of calorie-counting – increasing energy output through exercise is the same as decreasing energy input with a low-calorie diet. The overall effect is the same: you are eating less than you need and, no matter how long you exercise, as soon as you stop, you will put the weight back on again. The effect is most noticeable when the non-athlete performs bouts of strenuous exercise every two or three days. Any lost weight is replaced between one bout and the next.

The effect on your body's brown fat is similar to that of dieting: its action is temporarily switched off and if this inaction continues for any length of time, the brown fat becomes less and less able to fulfil its function. In the long term, the effects are as dangerous as low-calorie dieting.

The dangers of over-exercising

In women, exercise exhaustive enough to cause weight loss can delay the onset of puberty, cause amenorrhoea (cessation of periods), abnormal menstrual cycles, abnormal sex hormone patterns and impaired reproductive function, and the early development of osteoporosis (fragile bones). Male long-distance runners may suffer reductions in the male sex hormone, testosterone.

For anyone contemplating taking up the more strenuous forms of exercise, the advice from the *American Heart Journal* is:

> Be tested and have an exercise programme devised after clinical trials and tests on the heart as, although regular exercise will lower the overall risk of cardiovascular disease, there is a statistically significant increase in the risk of sudden death.

There are real risks if those who are not seasoned athletes attempt to break through the pain barrier, or as Jane Fonda puts it, 'go for the burn'. The pain barrier is the body's signal that its limit of toleration has been reached. Disregarding it is foolhardy. While seasoned athletes with their increased oxygenating capacity may be able to prolong their muscular activity before the onset of pain, the average person cannot and should not attempt to emulate them. The risk to health and even life is unacceptably high. Over the past few years there have been reports of significant numbers of cases of sudden death in healthy young men out jogging or playing squash because they disregarded the pain barrier.

There have also been a vast number of cases of broken bones, dislocations, and damage to internal organs, muscles, tendons and ligaments. A study from Japan cited a twenty-five per cent incidence of injury in those undertaking exhaustive exercise and these figures are confirmed in similar Western studies. The increase of sports-related injuries has been such that, had they been caused by a bacterium, it would have been classed as a serious epidemic.

Exercise-induced allergies – asthma, skin itching and urticaria – are also on the increase, as are cases of cardiovascular collapse and respiratory obstruction. While some conditions may be minor annoyances, others are definitely life-threatening. They typically affect teenagers and young adults. The usual trigger for an attack is running, but some patients have collapsed after only a brisk walk. It is not possible to predict an attack even among people with a history of such attacks while running. Even joggers who have been running for many years without incident frequently collapse. It is ironic that Jim Fixx, the inventor of jogging and author of *The Complete Book of Running*, himself died of a heart attack while out jogging. Current advice to joggers is: never jog alone.

In spite of the risks, or more probably because they are not made aware of them, many people adopt exercise programmes which involve sudden intensive exertion such as squash or aerobics.

The term aerobics means 'using oxygen' and it is claimed that aerobic exercise is beneficial because it increases the amount of oxygen in the body tissues. In fact, the demand for oxygen may increase to a point where it cannot be met, so that, far from increasing tissue oxygenation, aerobic exercise decreases it. Aerobic exercise has been demonstrated to cause a significant and continuous drop in blood pressure – a sign of cardiac fatigue. It can happen in as little as five minutes – and most aerobic sessions last for an hour!

And there is another consideration particularly where the overweight are concerned: by definition, people who are overweight are already carrying around extra weight. That fact alone means that they must already use more energy than slim people. There is a limit to how much more exercise someone who is massively overweight can do.

Athletes reach altered states such as 'the runner's high'. It makes them feel better and is a form of reward for their effort. The lower potential of overweight people means that they will be denied this satisfaction even if they do lose some weight.

Moderate exercise and sport do have a healthy social role. People who are part of a social group tend to have fewer health problems than loners. Members of religious groups, supportive families and clubs are also healthier, slimmer and more relaxed. However, excessive exercise is unnatural and can be dangerous. And don't be misled by the hype – athletes are not known for their longevity.

6

Are You Really Overweight?

Fashion, though Folly's child, and guide of fools,
Rules e'en the wisest, and in learning rules.
GEORGE CRABBE

Facts and fallacies about fat

After money, the topic that consumes people's thinking
most is their weight. People worry about how they ought
to look, whether they are too fat (they rarely worry that
they may be too thin), and about where their fat is on their
bodies. Then there are people who are already very lean
but who see themselves as fat and try to lose more weight,
running the risk of becoming malnourished. Some
anorexics may even die. Our perception of fatness is
subject to severe distortions and, according to obesity
researcher, Dr Alan Martin, who spoke at *Health Action
'92*, we also fall prey to a tremendous amount of
misinformation.

According to Martin, what is important is not total body
fatness but the way fat is distributed on your body. Fat in
different places on the body acts differently, metabolises
differently, and has different implications for health and
different body functions.

A French researcher, named Vague, described two
general types of fatness, the *gynoid* and the *android*. The

gynoid is typically female with a predominance of hip and thigh fat, and the android is typically male with excess abdominal fat. We now refer to the two as 'pear-shaped' and 'apple-shaped'. The difference between the two types is extremely important.

Fat cells do not behave the same in the region of thighs and buttocks as they do around your tummy. When fat is taken from these regions and put into test tubes, it may look the same, but that's where the similarity stops. Being very overweight can be a hazard to health depending where on your body that excess fat is. On your hips and thighs it isn't a health risk; it's upper body fat that is dangerous.

Abdominal fat cells give up their fat more easily than the fat from the hips and thighs. In other words, it is easier to lose the fat from your abdomen than from your hips, something that most women will know intuitively. It is quite natural that this should be so. Abdominal fat is excess weight in both men and women that serves no purpose other than to provide a store against lean times in winter. Fat around a woman's hips and thighs, however, has a completely different role: it is there naturally as long-term storage to provide energy and nutrients for a baby. It is designed not for pregnancy but for lactation. That fat has to be adequate to provide the energy required during at least six months' breast-feeding. Nature tries to preserve it. It is for this reason that upper body fat is shed much more easily than fat around hips and thighs.

There is a problem with weight loss from upper body fat: the faster rate at which fat comes out of the abdominal cells can lead to a fat overload at the liver. This is why it is important not to lose too much too quickly.

You probably would not have bought this book if you did not believe that you were at least slightly overweight. Models on catwalks, pictures in fashion magazines, and the slimming industry may have convinced you that you should shed a few pounds. But are you sure that you are overweight? Fads come and go, fashions change; how can you tell? This is an important consideration, as you should never try to lose weight if you are not overweight.

There is no doubt that to be too much overweight is not a desirable state, at least from a medical standpoint. Neither is being obese, as a rule. Even if being fat permanently is healthier than constant weight changing, it's not so easy to accept being overweight if your excess weight is ruining your quality of life.

One of the first signs that you are under stress from excess fat around your middle is shortness of breath. As fat accumulates, it crowds the space occupied by your organs. This may mean that you can't sit comfortably. While sitting your lungs have less space to expand, so your breathing is more difficult. But standing may also be a problem. Even if you are only moderately overweight, you are constantly putting an extra burden on your back and legs. Eventually, this can result in osteoarthritis. Too much fat around your middle means that surgery is more difficult; wounds don't heal as well or as quickly and infection is more common.

Even simple everyday activities become more difficult: lifting or carrying groceries, climbing stairs, bending, kneeling, bathing, and dressing. You are more likely to suffer from depression, nervousness, self-consciousness, and lack of self-esteem. It's all very well being told to accept your weight – but it's much more comfortable to be slimmer.

There are a number of ways to measure whether you are the right weight for your height: skin-fold thickness, body density measurement, height/weight tables, and so on.

The generally recognised definition of overweight is a weight that is above the acceptable weight for your height, and obesity is defined as being twenty per cent or more above the upper limit of the acceptable weight range. Having said that, however, we have to define 'acceptable'

as there are now known to be health risks associated with
extreme leanness. It is safer to be overweight than
underweight.

The acceptable weight ranges at present are those shown
on page 96. In these tables, however, women's acceptable
weight ranges are considerably lower than those for men,
and, as there is no reason why they should be, weights of
the two sexes are currently being brought into line. You
will also notice that there are no small-/medium-/large-
frame subdivisions. This is because these were always
artificial: doctors had asked for them and the acceptable
ranges were split arbitrarily into three. There is no
scientific definition of frame size. Unfortunately, the old
tables are still being used in current diet books and
slimming magazines, even though the concept of frame
sizes, for example, was abandoned as long ago as 1973.

The weight ranges for any particular height may seem
very wide as they cover a band of nearly 13 kg (30 lb) for a
woman of 1.45 m (4 foot 9 inches) to 20 kg (45 lb) for a tall
man, but there is no evidence that weight at one position
within this range is any healthier than at any other
position. A weight at the top is as healthy as one in the
middle or one at the bottom. Your weight wanders about
constantly over a few pounds and many people worry
quite unnecessarily about their weights. As muscle is
heavier than fat, a body builder with no excess body fat
can weigh the same as a person of similar height with
considerably more body fat.

There are a number of other methods you can use to
check whether or not you are overweight:

- Pinching a fold of flesh on the upper arm to gauge the
  amount of fat is a fairly realistic test, as it is more
  individual. But a figure of about 2 cm (^{3}/4 inch), generally
  regarded as the norm, still does not allow for individual
  physiology.

- Another useful measure is the Body Mass Index (BMI). For this you divide your weight in kilograms by the square of your height in metres (kg/m^2). If the result is between 20 and 25 you are an acceptable weight; between 25 and 30 is overweight, and over 30 is obese. This is the method favoured by clinicians.

- Alternatively, you can simply look at your face. If it is neither bloated around the eyes (which would be an indication of overweight) nor hollowed (an indication of underweight), you are almost certainly within the acceptable weight range. If you do not feel you are overweight, then you are probably not.

- There is one very good way of determining whether you need to lose weight for health reasons: if your waist measurement is greater than your hip measurement. In women, the distance around the waist should be no more than eighty per cent of that around the hips; in men, the waist should measure no more than the hips. Upper body fat is more of a risk than fat around hips and thighs. Fortunately, fat around the middle is easier to lose than fat lower down.

Height/weight tables based on Body Mass Indices can be found on the next page.

How much should you weigh?

Your weight is healthy if:

- You have no medical problem that's caused or aggravated by your weight,

- your family history doesn't increase your risk of a health condition related to weight, and your weight falls within the acceptable range for your height and age.

Age and height are the main factors that determine healthy weight. Within each range, higher weights generally apply to men, who tend to have more muscle and bone. Lower weights generally apply to women.

If indoor clothes are worn while weighing, their weight should be added. Estimated weights of indoor clothing are 3–4 kg (7–9 lb) for men and 1.8–2.75 kg (4–6 lb) for women.

IMPERIAL HEIGHT AND WEIGHT TABLES FOR MEN AND WOMEN AGED 25–59 YEARS

| Height | | Men Weight range (lb) | | Women Weight range (lb) | |
ft	ins	acceptable	obese	acceptable	obese
4	9			99–128	154
4	10			100–141	157
4	11			101–134	161
5	0			103–137	164
5	1	123–145	174	105–140	168
5	2	125–148	178	108–144	173
5	3	127–151	181	111–148	178
5	4	129–155	186	114–152	182
5	5	131–159	191	117–156	187
5	6	133–163	196	120–160	192
5	7	135–167	200	123–164	197
5	8	137–171	205	126–167	200
5	9	139–175	210	129–170	204
5	10	141–179	215	132–173	208
5	11	144–183	220	135–176	211
6	0	147–187	224		
6	1	150–192	230		
6	2	153–197	236		
6	3	157–202	242		

Metric height and weight tables for men and women aged 25–59 years

Height m	Men Weight range (kg) acceptable	obese	Women Weight range (kg) acceptable	obese
1.45			45.0–58.0	69.9
1.47			45.4–59.5	71.2
1.49			46.0–60.5	73.0
1.52	55.5–65.5	79.0	47.5–63.5	76.0
1.55	56.5–67.0	80.5	49.0–65.5	78.5
1.57	57.5–68.5	82.0	50.5–67.0	80.5
1.60	58.5–70.0	84.5	51.5–69.0	82.5
1.62	59.5–72.0	86.5	53.0–70.5	85.0
1.65	60.5–74.0	89.0	54.5–72.5	87.0
1.67	57.5–75.5	90.5	55.5–74.0	89.5
1.70	62.0–77.5	93.0	57.0–75.5	90.5
1.72	63.0–79.5	95.5	58.5–77.0	92.5
1.75	64.0–81.0	97.5	60.0–78.5	94.5
1.77	65.5–83.0	100.0	61.0–80.0	95.5
1.82	66.5–85.0	101.5		
1.85	68.0–87.0	104.5		
1.87	69.5–89.5	107.0		
1.90	71.0–91.5	109.5		

Prepared from data published by the Metropolitan Life Insurance Company 1983.

Fashions change

In primitive societies it is often fatness which is desired; in the West it is more likely to be slimness. Slimming magazines, women's fashions and the media portray the desirable woman as tall and thin. We live in a time when slimness is the fashion but it was not always so. Fashions change. Centuries ago celibate early Christian writers were terrified of women's flesh. They were frightened by their own lascivious thoughts, but put the blame on women. In an attempt to make women as sexless as possible, the Church urged women to fast. By the sixteenth and seventeenth centuries the fashion had changed dramatically. Rubens' paintings depict women who are considerably more curvaceous. At the beginning of the twentieth century it was still fashionable to be buxom, but by the 1920s busts were out and it was fashionable to be slim once more. In the 1930s the fashion changed to cuddly again – and back yet again with Twiggy in the 1960s. The Twiggy look has persisted.

However, we should be less concerned with what is fashionable and concentrate more on what is normal and what is healthy. In both sexes, body fat plays an important role: it fills hollows in the skeleton, the eye sockets, joints and neck; it cushions and protects internal organs and provides a reservoir of energy; it is fat that contours the body. When the body loses fat, it sags and shows the signs of ageing. Body fat is synonymous with the looks and actions of youth.

Women have more fat cells than men do. In a woman, up to twenty-four per cent of body weight should be fat; in men only about twelve per cent should be fat. Curves distinguish women from men. The woman's extra fat is both a natural and a normal phenomenon brought about by sex hormones during puberty. As well as having an aesthetic value, it is of biological importance, preparing the woman for motherhood. A feminine body is a curvaceous body. Why try to lose it? It is much the healthier attitude to be satisfied with what you have rather than continually try to change it.

Distorted perception and unnecessary dieting

There are many people who are not even slightly overweight, much less obese, who have been started by all the publicity on an unnecessary slimming programme that will ultimately have an adverse effect on their bodies' regulatory systems. Unfortunately, adolescent girls seem to have an exaggerated concern about getting fat, regardless of whether they are overweight or not.

Dr Nancy Moses and colleagues of North Shore University Hospital, Manhasset, New York, studied perceptions concerning weight, dieting practices and nutrition of 326 adolescent girls in relation to their body weight. High-school girls reported exaggerated concern with obesity regardless of their body weight or nutrition knowledge. As many as fifty-one per cent of *underweight* girls described themselves as extremely fearful of being overweight and thirty-six per cent were preoccupied with body fat. Many had a distorted perception of what was an ideal body weight. This was particularly noticeable among underweight girls; normal weight and overweight girls had better concordance between their actual and perceived ideal body weight for height. The team concluded that fear of obesity and inappropriate eating behaviours are pervasive among adolescent girls regardless of body weight or nutrition knowledge. In a society obsessed with body weight, even young girls who are underweight are dieting. Such inappropriate eating patterns are associated with many medical problems and poor growth.

Parents who are dieting also tend to put their young offspring on similar low-calorie diets. This can have devastating results. A growing child needs lots of protein to build body tissue. As a child's stomach is relatively small, he or she must also have a diet that provides lots of energy. Low-fat, low-calorie slimming diets are particularly dangerous to any child before puberty.

The milky way

The Jesuits say that if they have a child for his first seven years, they have him for life. Similarly, the way children are fed during these first formative years determines their eating patterns throughout life and will have a long-lasting effect on their later wellbeing and weight. Set good dietary patterns early, as trying to change them later is not easy.

It is noticeable that obesity seems to run in families: 'There's nothing I can do, my mother was fat, it's in my genes' is an excuse I often hear. But it is seldom true. One major reason for obesity is a mother's high carbohydrate diet while pregnant. Another reason that obesity runs in families is because children are brought up the same way their parents (usually mother) ate or were brought up. So if mother has a bad diet, daughter will usually have a similarly bad diet. This is how health and obesity traits are perpetuated.

Providing good nutrition for your infant should not be difficult. There is one product that alone will give her all the nutrients she requires for at least the first six months or more of her life. That product, consisting of all the essential proteins, fats, carbohydrates, vitamins, minerals and trace elements, formulated in exactly the right proportions, available when required at exactly the right temperature and germ-free, is mother's milk. Not only is it the right food for growth, it will protect your baby from allergies and gastric and bowel disturbances. Given free access to the breast, your baby will not overeat, taking only as much as she needs.

- A study published in 1990 showed that breast-fed infants are always slimmer than formula-fed infants at one year. Ninety-five per cent of obese people had not been breast-fed. Breast milk contains human Epidermal Growth Factor (EGF), a potent inhibitor of obesity. EGF is not found in formula milks or in cow's milk.

- For proper growth and brain development children under the age of two need fat and cholesterol every day – even if they are chubby.

Growing up

Childhood is a critical stage in any person's development. The way that children relate to their peer group is very important to them. Most important, particularly among girls and young women, is the way in which they perceive their own bodies. It is a sad reflection on our times that as many as two-thirds of young women between the ages of twelve and twenty-three believe that they should lose weight, even when most of them are actually already underweight.

Children generally follow the examples set by their parents. If mother is preoccupied with dieting, she will set an example that can profoundly affect the whole of her child's life. The pre-school years are the most effective period in which to establish healthy eating patterns. Habits formed at this time are likely to persist. It is important, therefore, to instil the right attitudes at this time.

Don't force food on your child. There is no need to worry about an apparent lack of appetite unless she is not growing as she should, both physically and mentally.

Do not reward good behaviour with food, particularly sweets. This encourages bad eating habits. It is much better to use praise. Similarly, do not use food as a comforter.

It also sends the wrong message to praise a child for

'eating it all up'. After all, she is only satisfying her hunger – a perfectly natural event. The danger here is that, if occasionally she is not so hungry and the praise stops, she will feel she has to eat more than she wants to earn the praise. This could lead to her overeating and, thus, to obesity.

The dangers of low-calorie slimming

If you think that you should lose weight, check with your doctor to ensure that it is necessary. This is particularly important if you are only mildly or moderately overweight and thinking of embarking on a crash diet, as you are at increased risk of arrhythmic sudden death on such diets. Then diet in a way that is safe. There is a serious risk of harm on very low-calorie liquid-protein diets such as the Cambridge Diet even under medical supervision. The 'yo-yo effect' of rapid weight loss, followed inevitably by weight gain, repeated over and over is far more dangerous to health than a high but steady weight.

Gallstone formation is usually thought of as a result of being too heavy but drastic very low-calorie dieting is much more likely to be the cause. Most diets restrict fats. But when a low-fat diet is eaten, the gall-bladder, which stores the bile used to digest fats, is not emptied. This means that bile remains relatively stagnant allowing gallstones to form. In a study of gallstone formation, conducted in America in 1989, obese patients were put on a 500-calorie-a-day high-protein, low-fat diet. Those taking part were very carefully screened at the start of the study to ensure that none had any sign of gall-bladder disease, but during only eight weeks, twenty-five per cent of the subjects developed gallstones. This is an alarming finding, as gallstones are not only painful, the operation to remove them is potentially life-threatening. The more one uses low-fat diets, the greater is the risk.

You should never try to lose weight if you are not overweight. If you are at your correct weight and maintain it without dieting, you have no need to diet. Having said that, however, this book will still be of interest as, if the principles of Eat Fat, Get Thin are followed, you will never become overweight.

PART
Two

7

The Eat Fat, Get Thin Diet

And ye shall live off the fat of the land.
GENESIS 45, 18.

If you are overweight and don't want to be, be under no illusions: you are going to have to make some changes to the way you eat – permanently. With most diets that usually means adopting a low-calorie, low-fat regime. As you know, this doesn't work. It doesn't work because it's unnatural and you simply cannot live that way.

The best way to lose weight and keep it off is to stop 'dieting' and eat naturally. That is what Eat Fat, Get Thin is: a perfectly normal – and, more importantly, natural – way of eating. It is a 'diet' only in the sense that anything you eat constitutes your diet.

Eat Fat, Get Thin is probably unlike any other diet you have ever tried. It's not low-calorie – you need never be hungry again. Indeed, you should not leave the table until your hunger is satisfied.

It's not low-fat either. There is no need to eat dry, unpalatable meals ever again. In fact, the more of the 'right' fats you eat, the more weight you will lose.

It is as well to be aware of what you are trying to achieve before starting this diet. What you are embarking on is an *unrestricted*-calorie diet. You may be eating between 2,000 and 3,000 calories a day. But don't bother counting them, they are irrelevant. You must, however, restrict your intake of sweet and starchy foods. You may find that merely cutting down on these foods is sufficient, or you may have to make a more conscious effort to avoid eating too much of them. Let your appetite be your guide. Eat as much protein and fat as your body tells you it needs. Historically people have preferred these combined in the proportions of one part fat to three parts lean protein.

No objection can reasonably be made to the Eat Fat, Get Thin diet. However, several arguments have been used against it in the past. The claim that a high-fat diet is fattening, or will lead to heart disease, has already been refuted. Let's dispense with the rest.

The fallacy of the balanced diet

There is no concept so dear to a nutritionist's heart as that of a balanced diet and it may be said by some that the type of diet advocated by Eat Fat, Get Thin is not balanced. To tell us what our balanced eating patterns should be, tables that divide food into groups are published in most countries. We are told that if we are to remain healthy, we must include food from each of these groups in our diets. Tables vary from country to country, but they are basically the same. This is a typical example of its type:

TYPICAL BALANCED DIET

Eat some food from each of the groups every day:

Meat, poultry, fish and eggs or dried beans, peas and nuts
Milk and milk products
Butter, or margarine fortified with vitamins A and D
Bread, flour and cereals
Green and yellow vegetables
Potatoes and other root vegetables
Fruits such as oranges, grapefruit and tomatoes

You will realise just how necessary a 'balanced' diet is when you consider that in many parts of the world large groups of hunters live quite healthily on nothing but a small part of the first group. It must be obvious from the evidence presented so far that people can and do remain fit on diets that are restricted to meat alone. And that observation is not confined to those one might call 'primitives' – the Eskimo and Maasai, for example. Similarly, the gauchos of Argentina, mainly descendants of European settlers, are near to being pure carnivores, as they live healthily almost exclusively on beef. Obviously, the 'balanced' diet so beloved of dieticians is not so important after all.

The truth is that a balanced diet is any diet that supplies all the nutrients the body requires, in the proportions it requires. A diet of fresh meat alone, if offal is included, can do just that. Liver, for example, contains four times as much vitamin C as either apples or pears; and kidney is nearly as good. Eat Fat, Get Thin, however, goes much further in that carbohydrate intake is not banned, merely reduced. It is, in all respects, a balanced diet.

Does a high-fat diet cause nausea?

Some may say that they find a high-fat diet nauseating. They associate the word 'fat' with blubber or greasy food. It is noticeable, however, that they usually have no difficulty eating fat if it is called 'butter' or 'cream', or served to them as bacon. The person who cannot stand 'greasy food' usually has no problem eating chocolate.

Strangely, although people have been professing to want leaner meat since the end of food rationing in 1954, the actual consumption of fat in Britain has been rising steadily throughout this century.

If you really cannot stand the sight of visible fat on a succulent piece of meat, you can avoid offending your palate by choosing foods that are high in invisible fats or the acceptable fats that you eat now. After a while you will find that you will come to relish the crackling on pork or fat on a piece of roast beef and you will be back to the ideal diet. At this stage fat will only make you feel nauseous if you try to eat more of it than your body wants. Listen to your body and fat will not be a problem.

Although at first sight this looks like a high-fat diet, and I have been extolling the virtues of fat, it really is not. There is no need to add fat to anything, for instance. Merely eat it as it comes: don't cut fat off meat, or drink skimmed milk. You may find that you are actually eating less fat than you did because you are not eating the cakes and sweets that combine fats with sugar.

Can it cause ketosis?

There is another objection your doctor may bring up which must be addressed. This is that high-fat diets can cause an undesirable condition called *ketosis*. Ketones are a class of compounds that are quite normal products of fat metabolism. They can be oxidised in the body to provide a source of energy. However, elevated levels of ketones – ketosis – can occur when there is an imbalance in fat metabolism. People unable to use glucose as an energy source – diabetics for example – tend to suffer from this condition. It is also found in people who are starving. Some low-carbohydrate approaches for weight loss actively promote ketosis by reducing carbohydrate to extremely low levels: less than 20 grams a day. I do not believe it is desirable, and have not found it necessary, to go to such extremes.

In the case of diabetes, the level of ketones in the blood is very high, often over 3,000 mg per litre. The level of ketones in the blood of someone on Eat Fat, Get Thin is insignificant compared to this, even lower than in a person who is fasting or on a low-calorie diet. In the clinical trials of a high-fat, low-carbohydrate diet, ketosis never proved to be a problem.

While there are clearly various levels of ketosis, they all have a common cause: dietary deficiencies of carbohydrate. Medical students will be familiar with the catchphrase: 'Fat burns only in the flame of carbohydrates'. Anyone who has studied nutrition will view this statement with some scepticism. History tells us that man, in many parts of the world, has lived, and still does live, healthily on dietary regimes that exclude all carbohydrates except the minute amount that is found in meat. The 60 grams of carbohydrate a day that are included in Eat Fat, Get Thin are more than enough to allay any fears.

Are cost and cravings for sugar valid objections?

Carbohydrate foods such as potato crisps, chocolate or bread and jam tend to be more readily available for snacks than meat and cheese. It is easier, therefore, to overeat sweet, carbohydrate-rich foods – and sugar is addictive. This can be a problem when you are eating what you are used to, and when well-meaning friends press such food on you. Sweet and starchy foods are also cheaper to buy. But anyone prepared to spend good money on unnecessary slimming clubs and magazines would be better advised to spend that money on good, wholesome food. It need cost no more than slimmers' membership fees. By eating properly, you will not get hungry and are much less likely to snack on sweets.

What if you're pregnant?

The ideal diet during pregnancy is the one advocated here for weight loss: one that has a high nutrient density with foods such as meat, fish, milk, and dairy products, and fresh fruit and vegetables. Eat too much carbohydrate and your baby will be fat. Dietary carbohydrates raise insulin levels. Studies have found that babies born to mothers with high insulin levels while pregnant are likely to be markedly obese by the age of six, independent of their mother's weight. It is not thought that insulin itself crosses the placenta from mother to unborn child. However, insulin produces anti-bodies that do. Once in the foetus, these increase glycogen and fat deposits, resulting in an abnormally large baby.

- Foods to cut down on are those that are low in nutrients and high in starches and sugars: sugar, sweets, bread, pasta, cakes and biscuits, and alcohol.

- During pregnancy there is an inevitable weight gain. This should be about ½–1 kg (1–2 lb) in the first ten weeks, 3–5 kg (6–10 lb) by week twenty with about ½ kg (1 lb) a week after that to the end of pregnancy: a total weight gain of about 13 kg (28 lb) over the nine months.

- If weight gain is substantially greater or less than this you should try to determine why. Excessive weight gain is usually caused by excessive intake of 'convenience food'.

Note: Please do consult your doctor before making changes to your diet while you are pregnant.

The Rules

Eat Fat, Get Thin is very simple in concept. Just follow these few rules:

- **Reduce your intake of refined carbohydrates.**

- **Exercise only if you want to.**

- **Don't try to lose more than 1 kilo (2 lb) a week.**

- **Leave the fat on meat.**

- **Eat a high-protein breakfast.**

- **If you are not overweight, don't diet.**

1. *Reduce your intake of refined carbohydrates*

You can eat as much as you want of any meat, fish, poultry, cheese, cream, butter, eggs – anything that is high in proteins and fats and low in carbohydrates.

You can eat as much as you like of green leafy vegetables: cabbage, brussels sprouts, cauliflower, broccoli, lettuce, celery, and so on.

Although there are some carbohydrate foods, such as sugar and cereals, that it is advisable to cut out altogether wherever possible, it is not necessary to stop eating fruit and vegetables, merely to cut down on the sweeter, starchier ones. For maximum weight loss, it is necessary only to reduce the amount of them you eat so that your total carbohydrate intake is no more than 60 grams (2½ oz) a day. Note, however, that the 60-gram limit is only a starting-point while you are slimming. Once you are down to your correct weight, it will be possible to increase your carbohydrate intake without regaining weight. You can also achieve a weight loss, albeit more slowly, merely by reducing your intake of the more carbohydrate-dense foods such as those listed below.

The foods that you should be most wary of, while you are overweight, are:

Sugar, sweets and candies
Bread, biscuits and pasta
Rice
Cakes, sweet pies, puddings and other sweet desserts
Jams, jellies, honey and syrups
Sweet, fizzy drinks, unless they are low calorie
Beer and sweet wines
Fruits that are tinned or cooked in syrup

Dried fruits
Root vegetables

You do not have to go through life never tasting these again. They are listed here because they are the foods with the highest carbohydrate content. As you get used to managing this diet you can reintroduce them. In the Appendix is a list of common foods and their carbohydrate content.

Some slimmers have difficulty giving up certain foods. Bread seems to prove a particular problem. You do not have to give up eating bread altogether (although it is a good idea to give it up if you can). Just cut down to a maximum of two slices a day, or substitute a starch-reduced bread. Instead of sandwiches for lunch, eat a chunk of cheese and an apple, or a bowl of cold meat and cheese with salad or pickles instead. If you like fruit juice at breakfast, drink grapefruit juice in preference to orange juice and reduce the amount. Breakfast could be, for example, grapefruit juice, fried egg and bacon, one slice of thickly buttered toast or fried bread, and coffee with cream and a non-sugar sweetener. This will give you a good start for the day, even though it comprises only about 18 grams of carbohydrate. Compare this with a small bowl of cornflakes and a 150 ml (a quarter of a pint) of skimmed milk: together these contain about 30 grams (1½ oz) of carbohydrate, which is half your daily carbohydrate allowance and you have hardly eaten anything.

2. Exercise only if you want to

Exercise has its place in a healthy lifestyle and has a social function. But as a means of losing weight it is a dead loss. Only do the exercise and sport you enjoy.

3. Don't try to lose more than 1 kilo (2 lb) a week

It is dangerous to lose weight too quickly, particularly if you are only moderately overweight. Be patient: on this diet you will not lose weight quickly, nor should you try to. If it took you ten or twenty years to put the weight on, it is unrealistic to think you can lose it all safely in a couple of weeks. On the other hand, you will not go hungry. It is the easiest of diets.

You may find that you do lose more in the first week or so. This is normal on any new diet. One kilogram (2 lb) a week may well be less than you are used to losing on a low-calorie diet but don't give up. Your weight will come down, safely and comfortably.

Start by restricting your daily intake to 60 grams (2^1/$_2$ oz) a day and see how your weight changes. This is only a starting point – you may be lucky and find that you can eat more.

4. Leave the fat on meat

Do not cut the fat off meat. Don't remove the skin from chicken, duck or turkey. Use full-cream milk in preference to semi-skimmed or skimmed; eat your fruit with cream if you wish.

5. Eat a high-protein breakfast (see Chapter 9)

It is essential that you start the day in such a way that your blood sugar levels are high and you will not have to snack between meals. A good old-fashioned cooked breakfast – eggs and bacon – is ideal, followed by, say, an orange. Ring the changes with eggs and kidneys or eggs and liver. Add tomatoes or mushrooms. If you can't face a fried breakfast, you could have cold meats, continental sausage, cheese, hard-boiled eggs, or fish instead. Never make do with cereals or toast and marmalade.

6. If you are not overweight, don't diet

If you are within the acceptable weight range for your height, you may not lose any weight on this regime, as it will not let your weight fall below your natural weight. If your weight is already in the acceptable range and you want to be skinny, this diet won't work. That's one reason why it is so much healthier than low-calorie diets that rely on starvation to achieve results. However, even if you are within the acceptable weight range for your height, there is no reason why you should not adopt the diet's principles as a precautionary measure. That will ensure that you never do become overweight.

The day's meals

I don't want to dictate to you what you eat. That is for you to decide. The Recipes section will give you some ideas, but below is a broad pattern your meals for the day should follow:

Breakfast

Select from:

fried bacon, eggs, kidneys, omelettes;

cold meats, ham and continental sausage (British-type sausages, unfortunately, usually have a high proportion of cereal filler and are high in carbohydrates. If you have British sausages, do not have bread as well);

kippers, bloaters, haddock either fried or stewed in milk and butter;

tea or coffee with milk or cream, artificial sweetener if required but no sugar; starch-reduced bread with butter or peanut butter, but not jam or marmalade.

If you have insufficient time to cook in the morning, prepare cold meats, hard-boiled eggs, cheese, etc. the night before. Or cook a meal the previous evening, when you are making dinner, and microwave it in the morning.

After such a breakfast you will not get hungry and you should not need to eat anything until lunchtime, but you should drink at least three cups of liquid: water, or tea or coffee with cream or milk, and artificial sweetener if required.

Lunch

For lunch you may eat:
  any meat with its fat left on;
  any fish, poached, grilled or fried (not in batter);
  cold meats;
  omelettes;
  cheese.
  Eat these with salad or a serving of green vegetables
  with as much butter as you like.
Follow with:
  an apple or other small fruit;
  cheese;
  coffee or tea with cream or milk but no sugar.

If you normally eat sandwiches at lunchtime, there are
some alternative ideas for take-out meals without bread in
the Recipes section. Some years ago I had a job that
required me to take my lunch with me. In this situation
most people opt for sandwiches, but sandwiches are made
with bread, and bread is high in carbohydrates. I made my
own 'sandwiches', in the form of two slices of processed
cheese, buttered and with a slice of meat, usually boiled
bacon, in the middle. It was a bit too rich and I did not
keep it up for long but it does show what can be done.
Now, in this situation I take a covered bowl of meat,
cheese or fish salad, or cold meat, cheese and pickles.

Dinner

Dinner follows the same rules as breakfast and lunch. If
you like an alcoholic drink with your meal, bear in mind
its carbohydrate content and treat it as any other food. Dry
drinks are recommended.

If you feel the need to nibble something later on, have a
piece of cheese, some nuts or a hard-boiled egg.

Low-carbohydrate Daily Menus

The Eat Fat, Get Thin diet is simply a matter of reducing the carbohydrate content of meals. You can eat as much meat, fish, eggs, cheese, butter and cream as you like, only cutting down on foods high in sugars and starches, such as sugar, honey, jam, bread, pasta and potatoes. Thus you do not really need special menus. Those given below are examples where the carbohydrate content has been calculated to give some idea of minimum daily amounts. Margarine may be substituted for butter if you wish. Do not use low-fat spreads.

Beverages with each meal: water, non-calorie soft drinks, coffee or tea with a little milk or as much cream as desired, sweetened with artificial sweetener if necessary.

Breakfast	Lunch	Dinner
1 cup grapefruit juice	beef steak with its fat	poached halibut
herb omelette	1/2 cup carrots in	green salad
2–3 rashers streaky	butter	cheese with 2 water
bacon	1 cup green beans	biscuits and butter
1 slice buttered toast	1 thin slice sponge	
	cake	
22 grams	*27 grams*	*11 grams*

Total carbohydrate for the day: 60 grams

Breakfast	Lunch	Dinner
half an orange	1 cup consommé	pork cutlets
scrambled eggs	roast ham	1 cup Brussels
2–3 slices streaky	cucumber and	sprouts with cream
bacon	tomato salad	1/2 cup carrots
1 slice buttered toast	1/2 cup fresh fruit with	small slice dark fruit
	cream	cake
20 grams	*20 grams*	*20 grams*

Total carbohydrate for the day: 60 grams

Breakfast	**Lunch**	**Dinner**
1 cup tomato juice	fried plaice	grilled beef steak
scrambled eggs in	medium serving fried	1 cup spinach with
butter	chips	butter or cream
salami	green salad	small portion
1 slice buttered toast	1 fresh peach	mashed potato
		2 soda crackers,
		butter and Cheddar
		cheese
14 grams	*30 grams*	*20 grams*

Total carbohydrate for the day: 64 grams

Breakfast	**Lunch**	**Dinner**
1 cup orange juice	corned beef	2 pork chops,
scrambled eggs in	tomato salad	including fat
butter	mayonnaise made	1 cup mixed
1 kipper	with cream	vegetables
1 slice buttered toast	cheese and an apple	¹/₂ cup fresh fruit
		salad with cream
20 grams	*15 grams*	*25 grams*

Total carbohydrate for the day: 60 grams

Breakfast	**Lunch**	**Dinner**
half a grapefruit	1 slice melon	asparagus soup
large portion of white	beef and vegetable	2 lamb chops with
fish, poached in milk,	stew, no potatoes	mint sauce
with butter	¹/₂ cup French beans	¹/₂ cup carrots
1 slice buttered toast	Brie or Cheddar	¹/₂ cup buttered peas
	cheese	small portion
		mashed potatoes
		fresh peach and
		cream
17 grams	*15 grams*	*30 grams*

Total carbohydrate for the day: 63 grams

Breakfast	Lunch	Dinner
1 cup tomato juice	oxtail soup	prawn salad
mushroom omelette	tinned salmon or	roast beef
2–3 rashers streaky	tuna fish	½ cup carrots
bacon	tomato and	1 cup cabbage
fried kidneys	cucumber salad	1 roast potato
fried tomatoes	potato salad	rhubarb crumble with
1 slice fried bread	fresh fruit salad with	cream
	cream	
17 grams	*15 grams*	*35 grams*

Total carbohydrate for the day: 67 grams

When your target weight is reached

When you have reached the acceptable weight for your height and age, you may increase the amount of carbohydrate in your diet or indulge yourself with chocolate once a week. But avoid the British brand-leaders. Not only do these chocolates contain so little chocolate that they don't deserve the name, they have an extremely high sugar content (sugar is invariably the first named ingredient). Better are the dark continental chocolates with seventy per cent cocoa solids. And better still (and cheaper) are some supermarkets' own brands, with seventy-two per cent cocoa solids. But watch the scales occasionally and if your weight starts to creep up, just reduce your intake of the carbohydrates again.

Aids to dieting

- To help you to stay with a diet, it is a good idea not to have any illicit foods in the house to tempt you. You cannot have biscuits with your mid-morning cup of tea if there are none in the biscuit barrel.

- When you shop, make a list and stick to it. If you are held up at the supermarket checkout, next to the sweets, don't be tempted.

- If you are going to treat yourself to a bar of chocolate at the weekend, don't buy it on the previous Monday – you are bound to be tempted to eat it sooner than you planned.

- Be aware of the signals your body gives you. If you carry on a conversation over a meal you may not notice when your appetite is satisfied and it's time to stop. Then you may eat too much.

- Respond in the correct way when your body signals that it's thirsty. Your body is telling you that it needs water – *not food*. When you are thirsty, drink water or a beverage that contains no calories. Having a sweetened drink, fruit juice or alcohol is one of the best ways to put weight on – without apparently eating anything! Try to wean yourself off sweetened drinks, even the low-calorie ones. Eating excessively sweet things is one habit you are better off without.

- If you like sweetened tea or coffee and don't want to use artificial sweeteners, try honey. Honey is as much a carbohydrate food as sugar but it is mainly fructose, and fructose is more than one and a half times as sweet as sugar, so you need only just over half as much.

- Resist the temptation to weigh yourself daily. Your weight will fluctuate from day to day (and throughout the day), and for women, throughout the month. Weighing yourself once a week is quite sufficient. When you do weigh yourself, do it on the same day, at the same time, and in the same clothes (or, preferably, no clothes) each time.

Conclusion

There are five important advantages to Eat Fat, Get Thin:

1. You can live on Eat Fat, Get Thin for the rest of your life without ever again being hungry. There is no stressful 'yo-yo' effect. Instead of starving the weight off, it gets the body to burn fat more efficiently.

2. It is very easy to live with and maintain socially. As all you have to do is reduce your intake of carbohydrates, you can eat whatever you are offered without having to disclose that you are 'on a diet'. You simply need to take a little more meat and a little less pudding.

3. With this diet, your weight cannot fall below its natural level. This is important. Being overweight may be undesirable, but being underweight is potentially far more dangerous. Serious risks of sudden death are associated with extreme leanness.

4. It is a healthy diet.

5. It is a natural diet.

8
Breakfast: The Most Important Meal of the Day

O breakfast! O breakfast! The meal of my heart!
Bring porridge, bring sausage, bring fish for a start,
Bring kidneys and mushrooms and partridges' legs,
But let the foundation be bacon and eggs.
A. P. HERBERT

French cuisine is admired the world over; the Chinese, in the West, are renowned for takeaways; the Italians for their pastas and pizzas; the Japanese for raw fish. Although, in gastronomic terms, England tends, it seems, to be thought of only in terms of fish and chips, the fact is that the English have given the world what is without doubt the finest and most important meal of all: breakfast.

In the face of a traditional cooked English breakfast the French croissants and Swiss muesli pale into nutritional insignificance; only the German cold meats, cheese and hard-boiled eggs, come close. For breakfast – a good breakfast, that is – makes all the difference: not only does it determine how well you will perform and how well you will feel throughout the day, it also plays a crucial role in determining whether or not you will get fat.

Whether you are trying to lose weight or not, it is better to take meals spread out over the day, rather than have one large one. The pattern that has been suggested for centuries is: 'Breakfast like a king, lunch like a lord and dine like a pauper.' In other words, the biggest meal should be at the start of the day, when energy for work is required, instead of the more usual practice of having it in the evening when all you are going to do is sit and watch television and then go to bed. It makes a great deal of sense.

The foundation course

Several lines of research have suggested that both children and adults get fatter and perform less well if they do not have breakfast. In 1989 there was an important meeting of the Forum on Food and Health that discussed a number of aspects of the various common breakfast meals. One of the contributors, Dr F. Belleisle of Paris, told of a study of French schoolchildren which showed that fat children ate breakfasts that contained, on average, seventy-five fewer calories and ate significantly more in the evening than their slimmer peers. 'Statistically,' he stated, 'the energy value of breakfast was inversely related to corpulence.' In other words, the less you eat for breakfast, the more weight you put on.

The average working woman and man needs some 2,100 and 2,800 calories a day respectively. If you are engaged in heavy physical work, you require more. If you are to spread out your calorie intake over three meals a day sensibly, therefore, you really should be thinking in terms of eating a breakfast comprising around 800 or 1,000 calories. And you cannot do that on muesli and skimmed milk.

Blood sugar deficiency

Your body needs over forty different nutrients to function properly. Unrefined full-cream milk supplies them all; refined sugar, on the other hand supplies only one.

Normally we eat such a wide variety of foods that deficiency of one essential nutrient seems impossible but there is one deficiency that can happen and when it does, even for a few hours, it can ruin your whole day: that is a deficiency of the blood sugar, glucose.

All body cells and the brain need energy to function. This energy comes from the oxidation of glucose or glucose and fat. Only when blood glucose levels are adequate can each cell obtain the amount of energy it needs.

Breakfast is the most important meal of the day because it determines what your blood sugar levels will be, not just for the immediate period after it is eaten, but throughout the day. That, in turn, determines how you will feel and act, and how efficiently you will operate. But just eating something is not good enough: for breakfast, quality is much more important than quantity. Eating too much of the wrong foods is as bad as, and in some cases worse than, not eating enough of the right ones.

If you have not eaten for twelve hours, your blood sugar level will be between 700 mg and 1,100 mg per litre, with an average at about 900 mg. This figure is known as the *fasting blood sugar* level. It depends on what and how much food was eaten at the last meal.

At the 900 mg level or above, energy is readily available but, as energy is used and the blood sugar level falls, energy becomes scarcer and you start to become tired. At the 700 mg level you will start to feel hungry and your tiredness will become fatigue. If your blood sugar level continues to fall, you become progressively exhausted, develop headaches, weakness and tremors in your limbs, palpitations of the heart, and nausea. It requires only a small reduction in blood sugar levels for your brain's energy supply to fall to a level where thinking is confused and slowed. As this process continues, you become depressed and uncooperative, irritable and aggressive. This is a natural reaction to starvation, programmed into all of us by our evolution: it is our body's signal to us to go out and kill something to eat.

In contrast, if your food intake ensures that your blood glucose is maintained at a level above fasting, you will feel on top of the world with plenty of 'go', be quick and alert, and have no feelings of depression or hunger.

Results of early breakfast studies

Many studies have been conducted into the effects of various foods and mealtimes on blood glucose levels. They have all demonstrated the importance of the breakfast meal, because it alone determines your blood glucose levels for the whole day.

In one study conducted in 1943 at Harvard University, glucose levels were measured for six hours after breakfasts that were high in carbohydrate, protein or fat. This is what it found:

- In the light of breakfasts today, the high-carbohydrate breakfast, which consisted of orange juice, bacon, toast and jam, a packaged cereal with milk and sugar, and coffee with milk and sugar, might seem quite good. After this meal, however, the subjects' glucose levels rose rapidly, but fell just as quickly to a very low level, causing inefficiency and feelings of hunger and fatigue.

- The high-fat breakfast consisted only of a packaged cereal with whipping cream. This time blood glucose levels rose only slightly and then returned to the fasting level throughout the period.

- The high-protein breakfast contained skimmed milk, lean ground beef and cottage cheese. This time blood glucose levels rose to 1,200 mg and stayed at that level throughout the whole six hours.

Unfortunately, in this series of tests, although it did show that a high-carbohydrate meal, which resembled a 'normal' breakfast, was the worst, neither of the others was representative of breakfasts in the real world.

Six years later another American test addressed this flaw. This time the subjects ate a variety of commonly eaten American breakfasts. To assess their relative influence, blood sugar levels were measured before breakfast and then at hourly intervals for three hours afterwards.

The findings, looked at today, are quite remarkable as breakfasts that gave the worst results are those that are most popular today:

- *Black coffee alone* was the first breakfast to be tested. This caused a drop in blood sugar levels, and feelings of hunger, fatigue, lassitude, irritability, nervousness, exhaustion and headaches that became progressively worse.

- *Two doughnuts and coffee with milk and sugar.* This meal caused a rapid rise in blood sugar, but it fell again within one hour to a low level, giving similar symptoms to the coffee-only breakfast.

- *A glass of orange juice, two strips of bacon, toast, jam and coffee with cream and sugar*, the typical American breakfast. Again, blood sugar rose rapidly but fell to a level below the pre-breakfast level within an hour, remaining low until lunchtime.

- *As the last, with breakfast cereal added.* The result was the same: a rapid rise followed quickly by a fall to abnormally low levels.

- *As the last, except that the cereal was replaced by oatmeal served with milk and sugar.* Again there was a rapid rise in blood sugar followed by a fall which, this time, was more rapid and to an even lower level.

- *The same again but with two eggs added*. This time, blood sugar levels rose and stayed up all morning, as did efficiency and a feeling of wellbeing. A similar breakfast replacing the eggs by fortified full-cream milk was also beneficial.

The effects of the various breakfasts on the subjects were then studied after they had eaten lunch. Those who had eaten the most protein at breakfast retained a high blood sugar level all afternoon. Where blood sugar levels had been low in the morning, after the largely carbohydrate breakfasts, however, levels after lunch rose only for a matter of minutes, falling to a low level that lasted all afternoon.

Both these studies showed that the amount of protein eaten at breakfast time was highly relevant.

Several similar studies have since been conducted. Where the foods eaten were realistic, the results were remarkably consistent: efficiency and a feeling of wellbeing experienced after meals is directly related to the amount of protein eaten.

Twenty-two grams of protein seemed to be the minimum for a breakfast to be effective. This kept blood glucose levels up for the three hours. Fifty-five grams of protein was required to keep the levels high for six hours. To put these figures in perspective, an egg contains between 6 and 7 grams of protein; an average rasher of bacon is about the same. Two eggs and two rashers of bacon, therefore, give you more than your 22-gram requirement. The best breakfasts of all were those that also included fat and a little carbohydrate. This was true of all meals.

Results of recent breakfast studies

By the 1970s, the practice of eating breakfast was declining, and cooked meals were being replaced by more cereal-based ones. As fat became 'unhealthy', full-cream milk on those cereals was replaced with semi-skimmed or skimmed milk. After the 1970s, therefore, trials aimed at testing the effects of breakfast on mood, cognitive response, problem-solving and obesity also increasingly used only carbohydrate-based foods. Results from these have tended to question the previous findings by purporting to show that high-carbohydrate breakfasts are best.

If these studies are taken alone, without knowledge of the previous studies' results, this seems to be the case. For example, workers at the Institute of Food Research and the University of Reading conducted a study of sixteen subjects given low-fat/high-carbohydrate, medium-fat/medium-carbohydrate, high-fat/low-carbohydrate breakfasts or no breakfast at all. This study found that not having breakfast did not have any marked detrimental effects. This suggests that breakfast is not so important after all, a finding that seems to refute previous studies, but this is not surprising when you discover that all the breakfasts were made up of varying amounts of white bread, margarine, jam, a sweetened milk drink, extra-thick double cream, maltodextrin (a commercially produced sweetener made from cereals) and water. The breakfasts were all seriously protein-deficient. Had they contained protein, the results would undoubtedly have been very different.

In 1995, Dr Ernesto Pollitt, Professor of Human Development in the Program in International Nutrition at the University of California's School of Medicine, conducted a review of papers published in refereed journals since 1978 on the differences in children's abilities after breakfast compared to fasting. He concluded, on the whole, that children performed better after having breakfast. But there were some notable exceptions. In some, breakfast made no difference to performance and in one study children did better when they did *not* have breakfast. It is significant that in all these cases, the meal was again almost entirely carbohydrate-based: cornflakes, semi-skimmed milk, sugar, wholemeal toast with margarine and marmalade.

Another study, conducted by Professor Andy Smith of the University of Bristol, sent completely the wrong message to readers of *The Times* on 5 April 1997. It reported a study of 600 people's breakfast habits and concluded that those who regularly ate cereal first thing in the morning had a more positive mood than those who ate other foods or had no breakfast. It also reported that elderly cereal-eaters were found to have higher IQs. But Professor Smith, speaking to the British Psychological Society, admitted that not only did they not look at the type of cereal eaten to see if one was any better than others, the study also provided no information about cooked breakfasts, because the diets of non-cereal eaters were not recorded. In other words, this study *looked only at cereals to reach its conclusion that cereals were better.* 'Better' is a comparative word. How can cereals be judged to be better if they are not compared to other foods?

Other reasons for having breakfast

The digestive enzyme, bile, is injected into the gut to digest fats. Until it is needed this bile is stored beneath the liver in the gall-bladder. Bile is not injected into the gut if no fat is present in food.

In the 1989 Forum on Food and Health meeting, mentioned above, a number of other aspects of the various common breakfast meals, as well as obesity, were discussed. Dr Ken Heaton of Bristol reported that missing breakfast could be a cause of gallstones. In a study of French women, he found that the women with gallstones had fasted for two hours longer overnight than those who did not have gallstones. This confirmed other studies which showed that a low-fat diet – and you can't get more low-fat than eating nothing – did not empty the gall-bladder. Fasting, he said, may turn the gall-bladder into a 'stagnant nesting ground for gallstones'.

Breakfast, for most people, is followed by a trip to the lavatory. This is caused by the 'gastrocolic reflex', which works best in the morning. Although a cup of coffee can set off this reflex action, the strongest stimulus is dietary fat. That may be another good reason for a fried breakfast. Anyone who is constipated would do well to cultivate the cooked-breakfast habit.

Conclusion

When you are thinking about slimming, *don't miss breakfast*. Studies have shown consistently that fat people eat smaller breakfasts and have bigger dinners than their slimmer peers. This evidence confirms that, in the effort to slim, large breakfasts and small dinners should be the order of the day. There can be no doubt that breakfast is the most important meal of the day. Miss other meals if you must, but never miss breakfast and never 'make do' with a slice of toast and a cup of coffee.

A typical breakfast for my family and me is one fried egg, two strips of streaky bacon, liver or kidneys and mushrooms followed by an orange and three cups of tea. I regularly travel into Oxford to read in one of the libraries, usually taking a bottle of water, and a piece of cheese and an apple to eat at midday. After my normal breakfast, however, I find that I can go until about 3 p.m. before I begin to feel hungry.

If you haven't time to cook in the morning or cannot face a cooked breakfast, why not hard-boil eggs the night before and have them for breakfast with cold meat or cheese?

Recipes

The breakfast recipes which follow are designed to fill and satisfy, to get you off to a good start. This is all important if you are to function at your best.

The ideas for lunches are aimed at the working man or woman who needs to carry a packed lunch to eat at the workplace.

As you only need to reduce your intake of carbohydrates to lose weight, dinners can probably consist of the foods you eat now with, say, more meat and less potato. Therefore the dinner recipes are gourmet ones for dinner parties or special occasions.

Breakfast recipes

As it comes at the end of a ten- or eleven-hour fast, breakfast is the most important meal of the day. Ignore it and the body may have to wait a further four or five hours. In this situation, the body cannot function properly. Not only will you be less energetic and mentally alert, such a long period without nourishment can harm the body's energy-regulating mechanisms. Any breakfast is better than none, but for peak efficiency you need to start the day with a good supply of nutrients.

Cold breakfasts, based on cold meats, hard-boiled eggs and cheeses, can be prepared the day before they are needed. If you enjoy a cooked breakfast, however, it is worth taking the little extra time it takes to prepare and cook one. An easy and quick breakfast is the traditional bacon and eggs. To fry these takes about ten minutes, only makes one pan dirty and contains no carbohydrate.

Frying

It is important to choose the right fat for frying as it must be able to stand a temperature of up to 200°C without burning or oxidising. It should also be free of water as this will make it spit. Clarified butter is by far the best for frying, but it is expensive, a cheaper alternative is lard. Beef dripping or other animal fats are suitable for frying but, as they tend to flavour the food being cooked, they should only be used to fry savoury dishes. Vegetable margarines usually contain a high proportion of water, thus they spit. There are white vegetable-oil based cooking fats which can be used for frying, and pure oils such as sunflower, and blended cooking oils which are suitable for frying. However, when heated, vegetable oils that are high in polyunsaturated fats oxidise readily, can cause free radicals to form and increase the risk of some cancers. It may be unwise to use vegetable-based cooking oils, such as sunflower oil, for cooking at high temperature: frying, grilling or roasting. Olive oil is not suitable for the high temperatures of frying. It also has a distinctive taste that may not go with the food being cooked.

If you use different oils and fats, do not mix them.

Most of the recipes below do not include bread or toast. If you include bread, reckon its carbohydrate content at twelve grams per slice.

The figure given for carbohydrate content is reckoned per person.

Poached eggs on toast

300 ml (¹/₂ pint) water
pinch of salt
4 eggs
2 slices white bread
butter
1 tsp yeast extract

Put the water and salt in an egg poacher and bring to the boil. Break the eggs into the poacher and simmer for three minutes until the eggs are set. Toast the bread lightly on both sides, then spread with butter and yeast extract. Remove the eggs and place on top of the toast.

Serves 2   *Carbohydrate: 12 grams*

Scrambled eggs

4 eggs
4 tbsp single cream
salt
white pepper
butter
2 slices white bread
2 tsp chopped chives
2 tsp chopped parsley

Break the eggs into a bowl, add the cream and salt and pepper to taste. Whisk with a fork until mixed.

Melt some butter in a small saucepan. Add the egg mixture and cook gently over a light heat. Stir constantly (or lift the pan occasionally) until the eggs begin to set, but are not fully set.

At the same time, toast the bread lightly and spread with butter. While the eggs are setting but still creamy, stir in the chives and parsley. Pile onto the toast and serve immediately.

Serves 2   *Carbohydrate: 13 grams*

Breakfast omelettes

These are basic omelettes with a variety of toppings. You could use the toppings listed below one at a time or combine them for variety.

Basic ingredients
2 eggs per person
1 tbsp milk or cream
salt and black pepper
butter

Toppings
streaky bacon
mushrooms
anchovies
tomatoes
shrimps with cream
cooked ham
Cheddar cheese
cottage cheese
herbs
flaked smoked haddock

Break the eggs into a small bowl, add the cream or milk and salt and pepper to taste, and beat until frothy.

Melt the butter into a frying pan and pour in the egg mixture. Cook over a moderate heat until it becomes firm.

When the omelette starts to set, spread the topping onto it and continue cooking until the omelette is set. Fold in half and serve.

Toppings. The cooked ham should be cut small before adding, the Cheddar cheese grated before adding. If cottage cheese is used, some may be mixed with the omelette mixture in place of the milk. The bacon should be cut into small pieces and fried first, the omelette mixture being poured over it.

Serves 1   *Carbohydrate: negligible*

Stacked omelettes

If making breakfast for four or more people, you might try stacking omelettes. First make up three or four toppings which complement each other. Make an omelette and slide it onto a plate standing over hot water to keep it warm. Cover with one topping. Make a second omelette and place on top, followed by another topping, and so on. Make as many omelettes as there are people. Serve by cutting the stack of omelettes into wedge-shaped portions.

Carbohydrate: negligible

Baked ham, egg and tomato

4 tomatoes large enough to hold an egg
100 g (4 oz) cooked ham
1 tsp chopped parsley
4 eggs
salt and pepper

Cut the tops off the tomatoes and scoop out the seeds and pulp. Remove the seeds from the pulp with a sieve. Mix the ham, parsley and pulp in a bowl with added salt and pepper to taste.

Divide the mixture and put into the tomatoes, pressing it well down. With the tomatoes in a baking dish, break an egg into each and sprinkle with salt and pepper to taste.

Bake in a preheated oven at moderate heat (190°C/
375°F/Gas Mark 5) until the eggs are set (about 15 minutes).
Serve immediately.

Serves 4   *Carbohydrate: 3 grams*

Poached haddock with egg

450 g (1 lb) smoked haddock fillets
600 ml (1 pint) water
4 eggs
black pepper
25 g (1 oz) butter

In a frying pan, cover the fish with water. Bring slowly to
the boil and simmer until the fish is tender but not
breaking up (10–15 minutes). Transfer to warm plates and
keep hot.

Break an egg into a cup. Stir the cooking water briskly to
create a whirlpool and carefully slide the egg into the
water. Simmer until the egg is set (about 3 minutes).
Repeat for the other eggs.

Cut the fish into 4 portions, sprinkle with pepper to
taste and melt the butter on it. Place one egg on each piece
and serve immediately.

Serves 4   *Carbohydrate: negligible*

Kippers and scrambled eggs

2 kipper fillets
4 eggs
milk or cream
salt and pepper
butter

Prepare the kippers: wash them well, cut off the heads and just cover with boiling water. Cook gently for 2–3 minutes, drain and serve with a knob of butter.

Alternatively, brush with butter and grill for 5–6 minutes.

The kippers may also be fried in lard for 5–7 minutes.

Mix the eggs with a little milk or cream, and salt and pepper to taste. Heat some butter in a saucepan. In it cook the egg mixture, stirring, until it is just set. This should be done while the kippers are cooking. Serve together immediately.

Serves 2   *Carbohydrate: none*

Fish omelette

This dish is a useful way of using up leftovers of a fish dish from the previous day. Any white fish may be used.

Remains of boiled white fish
1 tbsp milk or cream
4 eggs
a little white sauce
40 g (1¹/₂ oz) butter
salt and cayenne pepper

Remove any skin and bones from the fish and break it into small flakes. Melt a little butter in a frying pan, add the fish, seasonings and enough white sauce to moisten the fish. Keep it hot.

Slightly beat the eggs in a basin, add the milk and season to taste. Melt a full 30 grams (ounce) of butter in an omelette pan or small frying pan, pour in the eggs and stir over a high heat until the mixture begins to set. Then release from the bottom of the pan, put the prepared fish in the middle, fold the omelette over, allow it to colour, then serve immediately.

Serves 2   *Carbohydrate: negligible*

Egg croquettes

4 hard-boiled eggs
30 g (1 oz) onion
55 g (2 oz) mushrooms
30 g (1 oz) butter
30 g (1 oz) flour
150 ml (3 pints) milk
salt and pepper
1 tsp chopped parsley
pinch of grated nutmeg
2 eggs
55 g (2 oz) dry breadcrumbs
oil for deep frying

Chop the hard-boiled eggs and reserve. Prepare, chop finely and mix together the onion and mushrooms. In a pan large enough to hold all the ingredients, melt the butter and fry the onion/mushroom mixture until the onion is soft. Stir in the flour and cook for 1 minute. Pour in the milk gradually while stirring and bring to a simmer, while continuing to stir. Still stirring, simmer until the sauce thickens (about 3 minutes). Mix in the hard-boiled eggs, seasoning parsley and nutmeg. Stir over a low heat for 1 minute.

Turn the mixture onto a plate, flatten the top and cover with a second plate. Allow to cool. When cold, divide into 6 or 8 portions.

On a floured board, form into rounds. Beat the 2 eggs in a bowl. Dip the croquettes into the egg ensuring that each one is covered all over and, on a sheet of greaseproof paper, roll each one in the breadcrumbs.

Heat the fat and fry the croquettes a few at a time until crisp and brown. Drain and serve.

Carbohydrate: negligible

Lunch recipes

If lunches are eaten at home, their preparation and serving should present few problems. The dinner recipes which follow are equally applicable as lunches. These days, however, many people are away from home at lunchtime. This can make meal preparation more difficult. If you take your lunch in a restaurant or works' canteen, it is safest to choose meat, fish or cheese salads. Eat as much lettuce, tomatoes, coleslaw, etc. as you like, but go easy on the potato salad. You could also have a hot meal of, say, roast beef, plenty of green vegetables and a little mashed potato, but decline the Yorkshire pudding and go easy on the puddings: finish with cheese rather than a sweet. If you eat in a pub, and normally have a drink, bear in mind the carbohydrate content of the alcohol. Have, say, a whisky highball with soda, a vodka martini or a glass of dry wine – and restrict yourself to just the one.

If you normally take a packed lunch of sandwiches, however, it is not so easy. The ideas for lunches below, therefore, concentrate on meals to be eaten at an office or building site.

Sandwiches

Sandwiches should be used as sparingly as possible, and then be restricted to two slices of bread (carbohydrate content: 24 grams) at any one meal, spread liberally with butter. The secret is to ensure that what fills the sandwich is enough to fill you. The bread may be fresh or toasted.

Fillings
Cold beef, cut thickly with mustard and a slice of cheese
Minced lamb and mint sauce
Fried bacon and chopped pickled onions
Cheddar cheese and sliced onions
Cooked white fish with pickled walnuts
Grilled cheese on bacon
Cheese, ham and chicken slices
2-egg omelette with diced kidney and basil
Scrambled egg with anchovy paste and chopped watercress
Smoked cods' roes with tomato, lettuce and lemon juice
White fish with tomato sauce

Packed lunches other than sandwiches can be taken to work in covered plastic boxes and eaten either with the fingers or a knife and fork. These can reduce the necessity for bread and, thus, the carbohydrate content.

Finger salads

If the constituents of a salad are dry, they may be eaten with the fingers.

100 g (4 oz) full-fat cheese, (Cheddar, Brie, Gouda, Edam, etc.) or
100 g (4 oz) cooked sliced ham rolled around a soft cheese
  such as Philadelphia or
chicken legs or
hard-boiled eggs or
any mixture of the above
with a salad composed of, say, a stick of celery, 1 tomato,
  half a green pepper and 1 raw carrot.

Carbohydrate content: approx 10 grams

A similar meal, replacing the cheese with an individual pork pie, or egg and bacon flan, would have a carbohydrate content of about 20 grams.

Knife and fork meals

Salads to be eaten with a knife and fork can be more adventurous. The basis may be any cold meat; lamb cutlets, boiled bacon, chicken legs; fish such as sardines, salmon or tuna; hard-boiled eggs and/or cheese, together with a dressed salad (see Salads, p. 173, and Salad Dressings, p. 177). Carbohydrate content will be approximately 13 grams.

Dinner recipes

Dinner menus can probably be similar to those you enjoy now. All you may need to do is exclude or reduce the amount of potatoes, pasta, pastry and bread you usually eat (it is better to cut out pasta and bread), and compensate by eating more meat, fish, eggs and cheese. Eat these with about a cupful in total of root vegetables such as onions and carrots, and unlimited green vegetables. The recipes given below are for more special meals when entertaining.

Starters

Tomato sorbet

340 ml (12 fl oz) tomato juice
1 tsp Worcestershire sauce
2 tsp lemon juice
1 tbsp fresh basil leaves
salt and pepper

In a bowl, mix all the ingredients, and add salt and pepper to taste. Freeze the mixture in an ice-cube tray until it is firm but not hard.

Serves 2   *Carbohydrate: 6 grams*

Asparagus and peppers in mustard sauce

450 g (1 lb) asparagus, trimmed
1 tbsp tarragon vinegar
1 tbsp Dijon mustard
dash of Tabasco
dash of Worcestershire sauce
pinch of dried thyme, crumbled
pinch of dried tarragon, crumbled
salt and black pepper
$^1/_2$ cup extra-virgin olive oil
2 sweet red peppers, chopped

Cook the asparagus in boiling salted water until tender
(6–8 minutes), then refresh it under cold water.
Dressing. In a bowl, whisk together the vinegar,
mustard, Tabasco, Worcestershire sauce, thyme, and
tarragon. Add salt and black pepper to taste. Add the oil in
a stream, whisking, and whisk until it is emulsified.

Using a long-handled fork, char the peppers under the
grill, turning them every few minutes, until the skin is
blistered (15–20 minutes). Transfer to a bowl and allow to
steam until cool enough to handle. Keeping them whole,
cut off the tops and discard the seeds and ribs.

Divide the asparagus between two plates, garnish with
red pepper and drizzle the dressing over it.

Serves 2   *Carbohydrate: 8 grams*

Pork and herb pâté

450 g (1 lb) pork, minced
450 g (1 lb) lamb's liver, minced
1 large onion, minced
3–4 garlic cloves, crushed
1 tsp ground mace

1 tsp dried sage
¹/₂ tsp dried thyme
2 tbsp chopped parsley
generous pinch of grated nutmeg
salt and pepper
4 tbsp brandy
2 bay leaves

In a bowl, mix together thoroughly the minced pork, liver, onion, garlic, mace and herbs, nutmeg and season generously. Pour in the brandy and mix thoroughly.

Grease a 1 kg (2 lb) loaf tin and lay the bay leaves neatly on the base. After carefully putting two spoonfuls of the pâté on the bay leaves to keep them in place, spoon the rest of the pâté into the tin. Smooth the top.

Place the loaf tin in a baking tin and fill the tin with boiling water. Bake the pâté in a moderate oven (160°C/325°F/Gas Mark 3) for 2 hours.

Remove the dish from the water bath. Cover the pâté with foil or greaseproof paper and weight it to compress the pâté. Allow to cool and then place in the refrigerator to chill overnight with the weight still on.

To serve, turn out of the tin onto a serving plate so that the bay leaves are on top. Serve it either whole or sliced on a salad base.

Serves 10   *Carbohydrate: negligible*

Any pâté left over will keep for several days in a refrigerator or can be frozen for up to six months.

Soups

These days, tinned soups are easy to use and the labels give their carbohydrate content. To determine individual carbohydrate content, divide that figure by the number of people having the soup.

However, for something a little different, or if you prefer to make your own, try the recipes below.

Cold prawn soup
1 litre (2 pints) milk
2 tsp dried English mustard
1 tsp salt
1 tsp sugar
250 g (¹/₂ lb) prawns, cooked, cooled and chopped, reserving 2
    or 3 whole prawns halved lengthwise for garnish
1 cucumber, peeled, seeded and chopped fine, reserving 4–6
    slices for garnish if required
2 tbsp minced fresh chives

In a large bowl, whisk together the milk, mustard, salt and sugar. Add the prawns, chopped cucumber and chives and stir until well mixed. Chill the soup, covered, for 3 hours in the refrigerator. Garnish each serving with half a prawn and a slice of cucumber.

Serves 4–6   *Carbohydrate: 4 grams*

Cool cucumber and avocado soup

225 ml (8 fl oz) milk
2 cucumbers, peeled, seeded and chopped
1 avocado, peeled and pitted
2 tbsp chicken stock
2 tbsp lemon juice
¹/₄ tsp ground cumin

In a large measuring jug, mix the milk and sufficient ice cubes to measure 350 ml (12 fl oz) in total. In a blender, blend the milk mixture, half the cucumber, avocado, stock, lemon juice and cumin until the mixture is smooth.

Divide between two soup dishes and mix in the remaining cucumber.

Serves 2   *Carbohydrate: 14 grams*

Chicken and egg soup

1 litre (2 pints) chicken stock
100–200 g (4–8 oz) ground almonds
6 chicken breasts, chopped finely
6 eggs
salt and pepper
6 bread rolls

Bring the stock to the boil. Add the almonds and chicken and simmer for 15 minutes. While they are cooking, cut a hole in the bread rolls and scoop out most of the centre. Crisp the shells in the oven.

Strain the soup and fill the rolls with the chopped chicken. Keep warm.

Add the remainder of the chicken to the soup and purée in a blender. Reheat, adding salt and pepper to taste.

Poach the eggs. Place a filled roll with an egg on top in each of six soup bowls, pour the hot soup over and serve.

Serves 6   *Carbohydrate: 13 grams*

This soup may be used as a main course.

Fish dishes

Scallops in saffron

a pinch of crumbled saffron threads
2 shallots, minced
15 g (1/2 oz) butter
1 tbsp white wine vinegar
1 tbsp dry vermouth

2 tbsp double cream
50 g (2 oz) cream cheese
salt and white pepper
8 large scallops
plain flour for dredging
50 g (2 oz) clarified or ordinary butter
1/2 sweet red pepper cut into julienne strips
8 spinach leaves, washed and dried
2 tbsp grated Parmesan

In a small saucepan, cook the saffron and the shallots in the butter over a low heat for 2 minutes, or until the saffron begins to dissolve, stirring continuously. Add the vinegar and the vermouth until the mixture is reduced to about a tablespoon. Add the cream, bring to the boil and whisk in the cheese. Boil until it is thickened slightly (about 2 minutes), add salt and white pepper to taste. Keep the sauce warm, covered.

Dredge the scallops in the flour, shaking off the excess. In a frying pan, heat the lard over a moderate heat, until it is hot but not smoking. In it, sauté the scallops for 1–1 1/2 minutes each side, or until they are browned slightly. Add the pepper and spinach and sauté the mixture, stirring, for 3 minutes, or until the scallops are cooked right through. Pour the sauce into a gratin dish and spoon the scallops and vegetables onto the sauce. Sprinkle the mixture with Parmesan and grill under a preheated grill, about 100 mm (4 inches) from the heat until the gratin is just golden on top (about 2 minutes).

Serves 2   *Carbohydrate: 6 grams*

Trout with pine nuts

4 300 g (10 oz) trout fillets
white pepper to taste

plain flour for dredging
25 g (1 oz) clarified butter
100 g (4 oz) butter, melted
25 g (1 oz) pine nuts, toasted lightly
2 tbsp dry white wine
1 tbsp minced chives
1 tbsp minced fresh parsley
pinch of dried thyme
2 tsp lemon juice
salt

Season the fillets with the pepper and salt and dredge them in the flour, shaking off any excess. In a large frying pan, heat the clarified butter over a moderately high heat until it is hot but not smoking and sauté the fillets in it skin side up for 2 minutes. Turn the fillets and sauté for another 2 minutes. Transfer them to dinner plates.

To the frying pan add the melted butter and the pine nuts and cook over a moderate heat, swirling the pan until the butter begins to brown. Remove from the heat, stir in the wine, chives, parsley, thyme and lemon juice and salt to taste. Spoon over the fillets and serve.

Serves 4   *Carbohydrate: 2 grams*

Cold glazed salmon

½ cup dry white wine
4 basil leaves
1 tarragon sprig plus extra for garnish
1 sprig rosemary
2 sprigs celery leaves
2 shallots, minced
1 slice of lemon
1½ kg (3 lb) salmon
1 litre (1¾ pints) fish aspic (recipe below)

thin slices of turnip cut into flower shapes for garnish (keep
   in cold water to prevent discolouring)
1 hard-boiled egg yolk mashed with 1 tsp butter for garnish

Fish aspic
450 g (1 lb) white fish trimmings and bones
$^1/_2$ cup dry white wine
1 tbsp fresh lemon juice
1 medium onion, sliced
2 sprigs tarragon
2 sprigs parsley
1 bay leaf
salt and pepper
75 g (3 oz) unflavoured gelatine
white and shell of the egg (see above)

In a small saucepan, mix the wine, basil, tarragon,
rosemary and celery sprigs, shallots and lemon. Simmer for
15 minutes or until the mixture is reduced to about a
tablespoon.

Lie the salmon on a baking tray lined with a sheet of foil
twice as long as the fish. Raise the edges of the foil and
pour the wine mixture over the fish. Season with salt. Fold
the foil to enclose the salmon and crimp the edges tightly
to secure them.

Bake in the middle of a preheated oven at
190°C/375°F/Gas Mark 5 for 30 minutes or until the flesh
just flakes. Transfer to a work surface and remove from
the foil carefully. Remove the skin from the fish. Drain
the liquid from the foil and, using the foil as a guide, turn
the fish over onto a plate and skin the other side. Chill the
salmon, covered, for at least 4 hours or overnight.

Spoon a thin coat of cool but liquid fish aspic over the
salmon and garnish with the tarragon sprigs and turnip
flowers. Spoon a thin coat of cool but liquid fish aspic
over the decorations, and put a spot of the egg-yolk

mixture on the centres of the flowers. Chill the salmon for at least 2 hours and serve it with the chilled aspic chopped.

Fish aspic. In a saucepan, mix the white fish trimmings and bones, wine, lemon juice, onions, tarragon, parsley, and bay leaf, bring to the boil, stirring frequently to prevent scorching, and boil until it is reduced by half. Add 1 litre (1³/₄ pints) of water, salt and pepper to taste, bring to the boil, and skim it. Simmer the stock for 20 minutes, strain and allow to cool. Skim again.

Sprinkle the gelatine over the stock and add the egg whites, beaten to stiff peaks, and the eggshells, crushed. (Do not stir them in.) Bring to the boil, stirring constantly, remove from the heat, and let stand for 20 minutes. Strain through a fine sieve lined with a dampened kitchen towel, allow to cool and reserve 1 cup to coat the salmon. Chill the remainder until it has solidified.

Serves 3   *Carbohydrate: 2 grams*

Braised trout

2 trout
¹/₂ cup white wine
1 tbsp cider vinegar
pinch of ginger

Grill or fry the fish until brown and then simmer in a dish with the other ingredients until the fish flakes easily. Place on a warm serving dish, reduce the cooking liquid by half, pour over the fish and serve.

Serves 2   *Carbohydrate: none*

Creole prawns

4 slices bacon
1 medium chopped onion
25 g (1 oz) chopped green pepper
400 g (14 oz) tinned Italian tomatoes, drained, reserving
  1/2 cup of juice, and chopped
300 ml (1/2 pint) chicken stock
12 leaves Chinese cabbage
clarified butter
25 g (1 oz) chopped celery
1 rounded tsp plain flour
100 g (4 oz) tomato juice
1 bay leaf
pinch of cayenne pepper
750 g (1 1/2 lb) prawns)

Using a little butter, cook the bacon over a moderate heat in a large saucepan until crisp, then remove and crumble.

In the remaining fat, and on a low heat, cook the onion, celery and pepper until softened, add the flour and cook for a further 3 minutes. Add the tomatoes, reserved juice, tomato juice, bay leaf, broth and cayenne, bring to the boil and simmer for about 30 minutes, stirring, or until the sauce reaches the required consistency. Add the prawns, salt and pepper to taste, and simmer, stirring, for 3 or 4 minutes until the prawns are just cooked.

In the meantime, cut out the centre ribs of the Chinese leaves and chop them. Arrange the leaves, three to a plate, with the chopped ribs in the centre.

Pour the prawn mixture over the leaves and sprinkle with the bacon.

Serves 3   *Carbohydrate: 10 grams*

Prawn stuffed courgettes

4 medium-sized courgettes (approx. 100 g (4 oz) each)
butter
225 g (8 oz) prawns
2 tbsp lemon juice plus lemon slices to garnish
black pepper

Put the courgettes into boiling salted water and cook for 10
minutes. Remove and drain. Using a little butter, sauté the
prawns over a moderate heat. Slice the courgettes lengthwise. Pile the prawns on the courgettes and season with
lemon juice and black pepper. Garnish with slices of lemon.

Serves 2   *Carbohydrate: 10 grams*

Seafood au gratin

25 g (1 oz) butter
2 large red onions, finely sliced
black pepper to taste
250 ml (8 fl oz) fresh double cream
225 g (8 oz) large prawns
80 g (3 oz) red Leicester cheese

Use half the butter to grease four individual ramekins or
gratin dishes. Fry the onions gently in the remaining
butter until brown. Spoon them into the dishes.

Wash the seafood thoroughly, add it to the onions and
season to taste with the black pepper.

Preheat the grill to a medium-high setting.

Pour the cream over the seafood, followed by the red
Leicester cheese. Grill for approximately 5 minutes, until
bubbling.

Serves 4   *Carbohydrate: 2 grams*

Poultry dishes

Chicken and avocado salad

half a head of romaine lettuce, rinsed, dried and chopped fine
half an iceberg lettuce, rinsed, dried and chopped fine
small bunch curly endive, rinsed, dried and chopped fine
half a bunch of watercress, coarse stems discarded, rinsed,
    dried and chopped fine
6 slices bacon chopped fine
3 ripe avocados
2 chicken breasts (700 g (1 1/2 lb) in total), cooked and finely
    diced
1 tomato, finely chopped
1 hard-boiled egg separated and finely grated
2 tbsp chopped fresh chives
1 tbsp red wine vinegar
2 tsp Dijon mustard
1/2 cup olive oil
50 g (2 oz) grated Cheddar cheese.

In a large salad bowl, toss together the lettuce, endive and
watercress. In a frying pan, fry the bacon over a moderate
heat until crisp and remove with a slotted spoon. Halve,
pit and peel the avocados and cut into 15 mm (1/2 inch)
pieces. Arrange the chicken, bacon, tomato and avocado
decoratively over the greens and garnish with the grated
egg and the chives.

In a small bowl, whisk together the vinegar, mustard
and salt and pepper to taste. Add the olive oil in a slow
stream, whisking, and continue whisking until emulsified.
Stir in the cheese. Whisk the dressing and pour over the
salad.

Serves 6   *Carbohydrate: 7 grams*

A low-carbohydrate stuffing recipe for chicken is included on page 158.

Teriyaki chicken

2 tbsp soy sauce
$1/2$ tsp minced fresh ginger
5 tsp honey
1 tbsp medium sherry
1 tbsp white wine vinegar
1 garlic clove, crushed with $1/2$ tsp salt
450 g (1 lb) boneless chicken breast

In a bowl, whisk together the soy sauce, ginger, honey, sherry, vinegar and garlic paste. Flatten the chicken breasts between plastic wrap until they are about 15 mm ($1/2$ inch) thick. Marinate in the soy mixture for 20 minutes.

Transfer the chicken to a grill rack, skin side down, reserving the marinade, and grill under a preheated grill, about 12 cm (5 inches) from the heat, for 5 minutes. While the chicken is cooking, boil the marinade until reduced by half. Brush the chicken with some of the marinade, turn it and brush with the remaining marinade. Grill the chicken until cooked through (about 7 minutes), transfer to a cutting board and cut diagonally into 15 mm ($1/2$ inch) thick slices.

Serves 2   *Carbohydrate: 8 grams*

Chicken galantine

a 2 kg (5 lb) chicken
120 g (4 oz) ground pork
25 g (1 oz) butter
120 g (4 oz) dried figs, chopped

1 tsp ground ginger
2 tsp cinnamon
1 tsp salt
pepper to taste

Loosen the skin at the chicken's breast. Cut out the breast
and chop small. Sauté the pork in butter until tender.
Combine the chicken breasts, pork, figs, cinnamon, salt
and pepper, and stuff the breast cavities under the skin.
Skewer or sew to secure. Rub the chicken with butter and
sprinkle with salt and pepper. Roast in an oven at
180°C/350°F/Gas Mark 4 for 2½ hours, basting frequently
with butter.

May be served either hot or cold.

Serves 4–6   *Carbohydrate: 7 grams*

Pan-fried chicken with pesto

1 tbsp olive oil
4 boneless chicken breasts

For the pesto
6 tbsp olive oil
50 g (2 oz) pine nuts
50 g (2 oz) Parmesan cheese, grated
50 g (2 oz) fresh basil leaves
15 g (½ oz) fresh parsley
2 garlic cloves, crushed
salt
ground black pepper

Heat 15 ml olive oil in a frying pan. Add the chicken
breasts and fry gently until breasts are thoroughly cooked
(approximately 15 to 20 minutes).

While the chicken is cooking make the pesto. Process all the ingredients in a food processor or blender until smooth and well mixed.

When cooked, remove the chicken from the pan and cover to keep hot. With the heat reduced slightly, put in the pesto and cook gently, stirring constantly, until the pesto has warmed through.

Pour the warm pesto over the chicken breasts and garnish with fresh basil leaves. This dish goes very well with braised carrots and celery.

Serves 4   *Carbohydrate: 2 grams*

Duck breast with Chambord sauce

4 boneless duck breasts, about 170 g (6 oz) each
2 tbsp rendered duck fat (from making duck cracklings, see below)
2 tsp sugar
2 tsp cornflour
225 ml (8 fl oz) chicken stock
3 tbsp Chambord (black raspberry flavoured liqueur)
25 g (1 oz) butter
4 tbsp red wine vinegar
6 tbsp red wine

Duck cracklings. Remove the skin from the duck breasts and chop. Lie the skin in a frying pan, just cover with water, bring to the boil and boil slowly, stirring occasionally, until the water has evaporated and the fat is rendered. Continue to cook the skin cracklings in the rendered fat at moderate heat, stirring, until they are golden. With a slotted spoon, transfer the cracklings to paper towels to drain and sprinkle with salt to taste. Transfer the fat to a bowl to keep. The cracklings will keep for a week; the fat, indefinitely.

In a large frying pan heat 2 tablespoons of rendered duck fat over a moderate heat until it is hot but not smoking, and in it sauté the duck breasts, seasoned with salt and pepper, turning once, for 6 to 8 minutes or until they are just springy to the touch. Transfer to a cutting board and allow to stand for 5 minutes.

While the duck is standing, pour off the fat from the frying pan, add the sugar and vinegar and boil, stirring occasionally, until it is reduced to a glaze. Add the wine and boil until the mixture is reduced by half. Mix the cornflour in the stock and, stirring, add to the mixture in the frying pan with the Chambord. Bring to the boil, stirring and boil for 1 minute, remove from the heat, whisk in the butter until it is melted and incorporated and salt to taste. Spoon some onto four heated dinner plates, reserving the rest in a gravy boat. Slice the duck breasts thinly and arrange on the plates.

Serves 4   *Carbohydrate: 4 grams*

Turkey with balsamic vinegar and honey glaze

3 tbsp balsamic vinegar
12 tsp honey
350 g (12 oz) turkey cutlets, about 6 mm
   (¹/₄ inch) thick
75 g (3 oz) breadcrumbs seasoned with salt and pepper
25 g (1 oz) clarified butter or lard
3 garlic cloves, crushed
15 g (¹/₂ oz) butter
120 ml (4 fl oz) dry white wine
chopped fresh parsley leaves for garnish

In a small bowl, mix the honey in the vinegar until it is dissolved. Dredge the turkey in the breadcrumbs, pressing so that they adhere. In a large frying pan, heat the clarified butter or lard over a moderately high heat until it is hot but not smoking, and sauté the turkey in it, in batches, turning once, for 1 minute. Transfer to a plate. Wipe out the frying pan, and cook the garlic in the butter, over a moderately low heat, stirring, until it is golden (about 1 minute). Stir in the wine. Boil the mixture until the liquid is reduced to about 2 tablespoons, stir in the vinegar and honey mixture, and boil until the mixture is syrupy. Spoon the glaze over the turkey cutlets and sprinkle with parsley.

Serves 2   *Carbohydrate: 7 grams*

Poultry is usually stuffed and the stuffing in most cases is largely carbohydrate. Below is a recipe for a chicken stuffing which dates back to the fifteenth century.

Roast chicken stuffing

(for a 2½ kg (5 lb) chicken)

12 hard-boiled egg yolks
200 g (8 oz) parsley, blanched and finely chopped
110 g (4 oz) butter
pinch of ground ginger
½ tsp pepper
1 tsp salt
pinch of saffron (optional)

Mix together all the ingredients and stuff the chicken.

Carbohydrate: none

The egg whites may be saved and used to make shells for salads, stuffed with tuna fish, for example.

Meat dishes

Beef steak in pepper and macadamia nut sauce

650 g (1 ½ lb) beef steak cut into quarters
1 tsp Worcestershire sauce
5 garlic cloves; 2 peeled and crushed, 3 left whole and
    unpeeled
25 g (1 oz) butter
1 sprig thyme
1 sprig oregano
salt and pepper

For the sauce
1 sweet red pepper
1 tbsp beef broth
1 tbsp brandy
1 tbsp sour cream
15 g (½ oz) butter
1 tbsp chopped macadamia nuts

Rub the beef all over with the Worcestershire sauce,
minced garlic cloves and salt and pepper. Marinate
overnight in a covered glass dish. In a frying pan just large
enough to hold the beef, heat the butter with the thyme,
oregano and the unpeeled garlic cloves, on a moderate
heat. Fry the beef, turning it to brown on all sides, until
cooked as required. Transfer the beef to a plate, cover and
keep warm. Discard the thyme, oregano and garlic, but
reserve the fat in the frying pan.

To make the sauce. In a saucepan, mix the pepper and
broth and simmer until the peppers are tender (about 15
minutes). Purée in a blender until smooth. Add the purée
and the brandy to the fat in the frying pan and boil,
stirring, for 5 minutes. Whisk in the sour cream and cook

over a moderate heat, whisking until hot but not boiling. Whisk in the butter a little at a time until incorporated and stir in the macadamia nuts. Season with salt and pepper. Slice the beef and serve with the sauce.

Serves 4　　　　　　　　　　　　*Carbohydrate: 2 grams*

Caribbean beef pot roast

30 g (1 oz) clarified butter or lard
4 pieces braising steak, about 250 g (¹/₂ lb) each
3 tbsp rum
2 tbsp tomato paste
8 pimiento-stuffed olives, chopped
salt and pepper

In a frying pan, heat the butter/lard until hot but not smoking and brown the steak on all sides. Pour off the fat and add the rum to the pan. Simmer the meat for 20 minutes, covered. Stir in the tomato paste and salt and pepper to taste, and continue to simmer, covered, for a further 2 hours, basting occasionally. Remove to serving plates. Skim the fat off the juices in the frying pan and stir in the olives. Reheat if necessary and spoon the sauce over the meat.

Serves 4　　　　　　　　　　　　*Carbohydrate: 1 gram*

Beef goulash

60 g (2 oz) fat bacon
clarified butter or lard
1 large onion, finely sliced
1 garlic clove, crushed
450 g (1 lb) stewing steak, cubed
1 tbsp plain flour

1 glass red wine
150 ml (5 fl oz) beef stock
1 bouquet garni
salt, pepper and paprika

Chop the bacon coarsely. In a medium-sized saucepan,
heat the butter/lard over a moderately high heat. Add the
bacon, onion and garlic and sauté until softened but not
brown (about 5 minutes). Dredge the beef cubes in the
flour and add to the bacon mixture. Stir vigorously until
browned all over. Add the wine, the stock and the bouquet
garni. Season liberally with salt, pepper and paprika.
Simmer gently for 1–1½ hours. Remove the bouquet garni
and serve.

Serves 3   *Carbohydrate: 5 grams*

American meat loaf

2 onions, peeled and chopped finely
3 tbsp celery, finely chopped
2 garlic cloves, crushed
1½ tsp dried thyme, crumbled
30 g (1 oz) butter
2 tsp salt
1½ tsp pepper
100 g (4 oz) mushrooms, finely chopped
680 g (1½ lb) minced beef
350 g (12 oz) minced pork
100 g (4 oz) breadcrumbs
2 large eggs, beaten lightly
4 tbsp chili sauce or ketchup
420 g tin of tomatoes, drained and chopped
3 tbsp fresh parsley, finely chopped
3 slices streaky bacon, halved crosswise

In a frying pan, cook the onion, celery, garlic and thyme in the butter over a moderately low heat, stirring, until the onion is soft. Add the salt, pepper and mushrooms and cook the mixture over a moderate heat, stirring, until the mushrooms are tender and the juice they have given off has evaporated (5 to 10 minutes). Transfer the mixture to a large bowl and allow to cool.

To the bowl add the minced meats, eggs, half the chili, tomatoes and parsley and stir until it is mixed well. Form the mixture into a 175 mm by 250 mm (7 inch by 10 inch) loaf on a shallow baking tin, spread the remaining chili sauce over it and drape the bacon over the loaf. Bake the meat loaf in the middle of a preheated oven at 180°C/350°F/Gas Mark 4 for 1 hour.

Serves 6 to 8   *Carbohydrate: 9 grams*

Children love burgers and they also like pizzas. The following recipe is always popular with children but it is also just as popular with adults.

Burger pizza

680 g (1½ lb) minced beef
1 garlic clove, crushed
Worcestershire sauce
salt and pepper
clarified butter or lard for frying
thickly sliced bread (optional)

Topping
1 spring onion per burger, chopped
1 tomato per burger, sliced
1 slice Mozzarella cheese per burger
1 50 g (2 oz) can of anchovy fillets
1 black olive per burger (optional)

Mix together the beef, garlic, a dash of Worcestershire sauce and seasoning. Knead the mixture so that it binds together. Divide into equal portions – 4 for adults, 6 or 8 for children – and shape into burgers. Fry in a hot frying pan until browned on both sides.

Cut the bread into rounds just larger than the burgers and toast on one side. Place the cooked burgers on the untoasted side of the bread, top with spring onion, tomato slices and cheese. Add the anchovy fillets and place an olive in the centre. Grill until the cheese melts and serve at once.

Serves 4–8   *Carbohydrate: 15 grams*

Burgers need not be made from beef. Below is a recipe for lamb burgers and in the pork section is a recipe for pork burgers. Both are a little special.

Lamb burgers with béchamel sauce

Béchamel sauce
1 small onion
1 small carrot
15 g (1/2 oz) celery
500 ml (3/4 pint) milk
1 bay leaf
a few parsley stalks
a sprig of thyme
1 clove
5 white peppercorns
a blade of mace
50 g (2 oz) butter
50 g (2 oz) plain flour
4 tbsp single cream

Burgers
680 g (1 1/2 lb) minced lamb

1 garlic clove, crushed
salt and pepper
clarified butter or lard for frying
4 hard-boiled eggs, chopped
1 tbsp fresh chopped tarragon

Sauce. Prepare the vegetables. Heat them gently in a saucepan with the milk, herbs, salt and spices to simmering point. Do not allow to boil. Put a lid on the saucepan and stand it in a warm place on the cooker to infuse for 30 minutes. Strain the milk.

Melt the butter in another saucepan, add the flour and stir until smooth. Cook over a gentle heat for 2–3 minutes without allowing it to colour, stirring until the mixture (roux) begins to bubble. Take the pan off the heat and gradually add the flavoured milk, stirring to prevent lumps forming. Return to a moderate heat and bring to the boil, stirring constantly. When the sauce has thickened, simmer for 3–4 minutes beating briskly. At this point, re-season if required. Add the cream while the sauce is still at the boil and remove immediately from the heat. Do not allow it to boil once the cream has been added.

Burgers. Mix the lamb, garlic and plenty of seasoning, knead together so that it binds, divide into equal amounts – 4 for adults, 6 or 8 for children – and shape into burgers. Fry in a hot pan until browned on both sides.

Arrange the burgers on a serving dish then pour some of the sauce over and serve immediately. The remaining sauce may be served in a sauce boat.

Serves 4 adults   *Carbohydrate: 6 grams*

Lamb chops in lemon caper sauce

two 40 mm (1½ inch) thick lamb chops or 4 smaller ones
15 g (½ oz) butter

1 tsp grated lemon zest
1 tsp bottled capers, drained
1 tbsp lemon juice

Sprinkle the lamb chops with salt and pepper and grill them under a preheated grill, about 100 mm (4 inches) from the heat for 6 minutes (less for the smaller chops). Turn over and grill for a further 4 minutes for medium-rare meat. Let them stand for 5 minutes.

While the chops are standing, in a small saucepan melt the butter and stir in the zest, the capers, lemon juice and salt and pepper to taste.

Transfer the chops to plates and pour the sauce over them.

Serves 2   *Carbohydrate: negligible*

Herbed roast leg of lamb with onions

60 g (2 oz) Dijon mustard
1 large garlic clove crushed to a paste with $^1/_4$ tsp salt
$^1/_2$ tbsp finely chopped fresh rosemary (or 1 tsp dried, crumbled) plus a fresh sprig for garnish
$^1/_2$ tbsp finely chopped fresh thyme (or 1 tsp dried, crumbled) plus a fresh sprig for garnish
1 tbsp soy sauce
75 ml (2 fl oz) dry white wine
salt and pepper
2 tbsp olive oil
3.5 kg (8 lb) leg of lamb, pelvic bone removed and tied
1 kg (2 lb) small onions, blanched in boiling water for 2 minutes, drained and peeled
2 large carrots cut into 12 mm ($^1/_2$ inch) pieces

Gravy
1 cup red wine

2 cups beef broth
30 g (1 oz) butter, softened
2 tbsp plain flour
salt and pepper

In a small bowl, whisk together the mustard, garlic, rosemary, thyme, soy sauce, and wine, adding salt and pepper to taste. Add 1 tablespoon of olive oil in a stream, whisking, and continue whisking until the mixture is thoroughly combined. Brush the lamb generously on all sides with some of the mixture, reserving the rest, and let it marinate in a lightly larded roasting pan, covered and chilled, for at least 6 hours and preferably overnight.

Let the lamb return to room temperature and brush it with the rest of the mustard mixture. In a bowl, toss the onions in the rest of the oil, add them and the carrots to the baking pan and roast them with the lamb in the middle of a preheated oven at 230°C/450°F/Gas Mark 8 for 15 minutes. Reduce the temperature to 180°C/350°F/Gas Mark 4 and roast, stirring the vegetables occasionally, for 1 hour 15 minutes, for medium-rare meat. Transfer the lamb to a platter and let stand for 20 minutes. Transfer the onions with a slotted spoon to a serving dish, leaving the carrots in the pan, and keep them warm, covered.

To make the gravy. Pour off the fat from the pan, reserving the other juices. Transfer the juices and carrots to a saucepan and add the wine. Boil the mixture until reduced by half and mash the carrots. Add the broth and bring to the boil. In a small bowl knead together the butter and flour until combined well and add to the mixture a little at a time, whisking. Add salt and pepper to taste. Simmer the gravy, whisking occasionally, until thickened (about 3 minutes).

Garnish the lamb with thyme and rosemary sprigs.

Serves 8   *Carbohydrate: 2 grams*

Lamb chops with mint vinegar sauce

12 small lamb chops
1 garlic clove, halved across
$^1/_2$ tsp dried thyme, crumbled
white pepper to taste

Sauce
2 tbsp white wine vinegar
2 tbsp granulated sugar
2 tbsp fresh spearmint leaves, minced

For the sauce. In a small saucepan, mix the vinegar and
sugar and cook over a moderate heat, stirring, until the
sugar has dissolved. Stir in the spearmint and let the
mixture cool. Season the sauce with salt and pepper to
taste and transfer to a bowl.

Rub the chops with the cut sides of the garlic and
sprinkle them on both sides with the thyme and pepper.
Sauté in a larded pan over a moderately high heat on both
sides for about 2 minutes, for medium-rare meat. Serve
with the sauce.

Serves 4 or 6   *Carbohydrate: 8 or 6 grams*

Minced lamb with fennel

2 medium onions, chopped
25 g (1 oz) butter
500 g (1 lb 2 oz) lamb mince
1 medium bulb fennel, sliced thinly
1 tbsp ground coriander
1 tsp cumin seeds
440 g (1 tin) chopped tomatoes
2 tbsp tomato purée
1 tbsp fresh parsley

Fry the onion in the butter until it is brown. Add the lamb and cook until that is browned. Add the fennel and spices. Lower the heat. Stir in the rest of the ingredients, partially cover and simmer for 25 minutes.

Serves 4   *Carbohydrate: 12 grams*

Chicken satay

1 medium onion, minced
1 garlic clove, crushed
1 tsp fresh coriander, chopped
1 tsp fresh ginger, minced and peeled
1 tbsp rice wine vinegar
1 tbsp vegetable oil
1 tsp Chinese chili paste
900 g (2 lb) chicken cut into 20 mm (³/₄ inch) cubes
ten 260 mm (10 inch) wooden skewers soaked in cold water
   for 30 minutes

Sauce
12 g (¹/₂ oz butter)
25 g (1 oz) dry-roasted peanuts, crushed
3 shallots, chopped
1 garlic clove, crushed
¹/₂ tsp shrimp paste
¹/₂ tsp Chinese chili paste
1 tbsp fresh lemon juice

In a shallow dish, mix the onion, garlic, coriander, ginger, oil, vinegar and chili. Add the chicken, stirring to coat it with the marinade and let it marinate, covered, overnight.
   Sauce. In a saucepan heat the butter and cook the peanuts, shallots, garlic and shrimp paste, stirring for 1 minute or until the mixture thickens. Add the chili paste and lemon juice and 1¹/₂ cups of water, and simmer for 5–7

minutes, or until thickened, stirring occasionally. Season with salt and pepper to taste.

Thread the chicken onto the skewers, grill for 10 minutes on each side and transfer to a serving plate. Pour the sauce over the chicken. Makes about 10 satays.

Serves 4–5   *Carbohydrate: 5 grams*

Egg and Cheese

Cheese and tomato soufflés

25 g (1 oz) butter
1 tbsp plain flour
275 ml (¹/₂ pint) milk
2 tbsp tomato paste
1 cup grated Swiss cheese
2 tbsp grated Parmesan cheese
cayenne pepper
salt
3 large eggs, separated
1 tbsp medium sherry

In a saucepan, melt the butter over a low heat, stir in the flour and cook the roux, stirring, for 3 minutes. Bring the milk to the boil. Remove the roux pan from the heat and add the scalded milk, in a stream, whisking vigorously until the mixture is thick and smooth. Simmer the sauce for 3–4 minutes, or until thickened, and whisk in the tomato paste, cheeses, cayenne pepper and salt to taste. Continue whisking until the cheeses have melted. Remove from the heat and whisk in the egg yolks, one at a time, beating each well in. Transfer to a bowl to cool.

In a bowl, whisk the egg whites with a pinch of salt, until they maintain soft peaks, add the sherry and beat the mixture until it maintains stiff peaks. Fold the egg white mixture into the cheese mixture gently but thoroughly, transfer to 6 buttered ramekins, and bake the soufflés in the middle of a preheated oven at 200°C/400°F/Gas Mark 6 for 25–30 minutes, or until cooked through.

Serves 6   *Carbohydrate: 4 grams*

Blue cheese omelette

60 g (2 oz) blue cheese, crumbled
2 tbsp double cream
4 large eggs
large pinch each of salt and pepper
25 g (1 oz) butter

In a bowl, stir together the cheese and the cream. In another bowl, beat the eggs with a fork and stir in the salt and pepper. In a frying pan, heat the butter over a moderate heat until the foam begins to subside, add the egg mixture and cook, covered.

When the top begins to firm, spoon the cheese mixture over the omelette and cook until the cheese thickens (about 2 minutes). Fold the omelette in half over the cheese filling and serve.

Serves 2   *Carbohydrate: none*

Savoury cheesecake

2 tbsp grated Parmesan cheese
2 tbsp fine dry breadcrumbs
425 ml (³/₄ pint) double cream
250 g (8 oz) blue cheese, crumbled
680 g (1¹/₂ lb) cream cheese, cut into pieces and softened
4 large eggs

In a bowl, mix well with the Parmesan and breadcrumbs and coat the inside of a 23 cm (9 inch) cake tin. In a saucepan scald the cream.

In a large bowl, with an electric whisk, blend the blue cheese with 2 tablespoons of the cream until the mixture is smooth, add half the cream cheese and beat until it is smooth. Beat in the remaining cream and beat until smooth. Beat in the eggs, one at a time, and continue beating until the mixture is smooth. Pour into the prepared cake tin.

Bake the cheesecake in the bottom of a preheated oven at 160°C/325°F/Gas Mark 3, until the centre is just firm (about 1 hour 15 minutes).

Let the cheesecake cool completely, preferably overnight. Turn out and slice thinly.

Serves 6–8   *Carbohydrate: negligible*

Baked stuffed eggs

60 g (2 oz) butter
2 shallots, minced
6 mushrooms, finely chopped
2 tbsp milk
2 tbsp single cream
2 tbsp dry white wine
6 large hard-boiled eggs
salt and pepper

Sauce
25 g (1 oz) butter
2 tbsp plain flour
425 ml (³/₄ pint) milk, scalded
140 g (5 oz) Gruyère cheese, grated
1 egg yolk

In a frying pan, heat the butter until hot and sauté the shallots over a moderate heat, stirring occasionally, until softened (about 4 minutes). Add the mushrooms, milk, cream and wine, and simmer the mixture, stirring occasionally, for 15 minutes. Allow to cool.

Halve the eggs lengthwise, remove the yolks and crumble them in a bowl. Stir in the mushroom mixture and combine well. Add salt and pepper to taste. Divide the mixture between the egg whites, place one half on top of another and re-form each egg into its original shape.

Sauce. In a saucepan, melt the butter over a low heat, stir in the flour and cook over a moderate heat, stirring, for 3 minutes. Remove from the heat and add the scalded milk in a stream, whisking, and cook the mixture, whisking vigorously, until it is smooth and has thickened. Remove from the heat and stir in half the Gruyère, egg yolk and salt and pepper to taste. Spoon one third of the sauce into an oven-proof serving dish, just large enough to hold the eggs, cover them with the remaining sauce, sprinkle with the remaining half of the Gruyère, and bake them in the upper third of a pre-heated very hot oven at 260°C/500°F/Gas Mark 10, until the cheese is bubbly and browned slightly (about 10 minutes).

Serves 6   *Carbohydrate: 7 grams*

Eggs with anchovies

12 eggs
85 g (3 oz) butter
30 g (1 oz) pistachio nuts, shelled and crushed
4 anchovies, crushed
3–4 tbsp beef or lamb stock, or white wine
lettuce leaves

Scramble the eggs in the butter over a low heat while stirring in the nuts. Purée the anchovies in the stock and stir into the eggs as they begin to harden. Serve on the lettuce leaves or with a salad.

Serves 6   *Carbohydrate: negligible*

Salads

The following salads are not designed to be eaten alone but as accompaniments to cold meats, fish etc.

Mushroom salad

3 tbsp olive oil
1¹/₂ tbsp plain yoghurt
1¹/₂ tbsp lemon juice
3 tbsp sour cream
1 tsp minced shallot or onion
1 large garlic clove, crushed to a pulp
¹/₂ tsp salt
2 tbsp minced fresh parsley
450 g (1 lb) button mushrooms
ground white pepper

In a bowl, mix together the oil, yoghurt, lemon juice, sour cream, shallot, garlic, salt and parsley. Toss the mushrooms in the mixture gently but thoroughly. Season with salt and pepper.

Serves 4–6   *Carbohydrate: 4 grams*

Chicory and watercress salad

1 tbsp sherry (or white wine) vinegar
¹/₂ tsp Dijon mustard
2 tbsp walnut oil
1 tbsp olive oil

1 large bunch watercress, rinsed and dried, coarse stems discarded
1 chicon of French or Italian chicory, rinsed and dried

Whisk together the vinegar and mustard. Add the oils in a stream, whisking, and add salt and pepper to taste. Whisk until emulsified. Toss the watercress and chicory in the dressing.

Serves 4   *Carbohydrate: 2 grams*

Blue cheese and walnut winter salad

1 small head radicchio lettuce, separated, rinsed, dried and torn into small pieces
1 small head cos lettuce, separated, rinsed, dried and torn into small pieces
1 bunch watercress, rinsed and dried, coarse stems discarded
1 endive, leaves separated and torn in half

Dressing
3 shallots, peeled
2 tbsp white wine vinegar
$1/2$ tsp salt
$1/4$ tsp pepper
$1/2$ cup extra virgin olive oil
1 tsp walnut oil
36 walnut halves, toasted
250 g ($1/2$ lb) blue cheese, crumbled

Toss together the radicchio and cos lettuce, watercress and endive.
    Make the dressing. Under a moderately high heat, grill the shallots on each side until golden and fragrant (about 5–6 minutes) Cool, then chop fine. In a bowl, combine the

shallots, vinegar, salt and pepper, add the oils in a stream, whisking, and whisk until the dressing has emulsified. Pour the dressing over the salad and add the walnuts and cheese. Toss well to combine and serve.

Serves 4–6   *Carbohydrate: 13 grams*

Parmesan and anchovy salad

3 garlic cloves
3 anchovy fillets, drained and mashed
2 large egg yolks
2 tsp white wine vinegar
2 tsp balsamic vinegar
1¹/₂ tsp Dijon mustard
1 tsp Worcestershire sauce
¹/₄ tsp salt
1¹/₂ tsp lime juice
³/₄ cup extra virgin olive oil
2 heads of romaine lettuce, rinsed, dried and torn into strips
40 g (1¹/₂ oz) Parmesan cheese, grated

Crush the garlic and mash with the anchovies to form a paste. Whisk the paste with the egg yolks, vinegars, mustard, Worcestershire sauce, salt and lime juice. Add the oil in a stream and whisk until emulsified.

Toss the romaine lettuce and Parmesan cheese in a bowl, add the dressing and toss until combined well.

Serves 4–6   *Carbohydrate: 3 grams*

Watercress and radicchio salad

1 tbsp white wine vinegar
¹/₂ tsp Dijon mustard
2 tsp fresh parsley leaves, chopped
salt and pepper

1 tbsp extra virgin olive oil

2 bunches watercress, washed, dried and separated into sprigs

2 small heads of radicchio lettuce, washed, dried and finely shredded

3 spring onions, sliced

175 g (6 oz) Parmesan cheese, grated

In a small bowl, whisk together the vinegar, mustard, parsley, salt and pepper. Add the oil in a stream, whisking the dressing until it has emulsified.

In a salad bowl, toss together the watercress, radicchio lettuce and spring onions. Pour the dressing over the salad and toss well. Cover with Parmesan cheese.

Serves 8   *Carbohydrate: 3 grams*

Mushroom, radish and endive salad

$^1/_2$ tsp Dijon mustard

1 tbsp red wine vinegar

2 tbsp extra virgin olive oil

8 leaves soft lettuce, rinsed and dried

4 radishes, trimmed and thinly sliced

4 button mushrooms, thinly sliced

1 large endive, trimmed and cut across into 6 mm ($^1/_4$ inch) slices

one sprig of fresh parsley leaves

salt and pepper

In a salad bowl, whisk together the mustard, vinegar and salt to taste. Add the oil a little at a time, whisking, and whisk the dressing until emulsified. Add the lettuce, radishes, mushrooms, endive, parsley and pepper. Toss the salad to coat with the dressing.

Serves 2   *Carbohydrate: 5 grams*

Salad dressings

Mayonnaise

2 large egg yolks
2 tsp wine vinegar
1 tsp Dijon mustard (or to taste)
$^1/_4$ tsp salt
white pepper
$1^1/_2$ cups olive oil or vegetable oil
fresh lemon juice (to taste)
single cream

Warm a mixing bowl with hot water and dry well. In the bowl, combine the egg yolks, 1 teaspoon of vinegar, the mustard, salt and pepper. Beat or whisk vigorously until the mixture is well combined. Add half a cup of oil, drop by drop, beating constantly. Add the remaining teaspoon of vinegar and the remaining cup of oil in a stream, whisking constantly. Add the lemon juice, white pepper and salt to taste and thin with cream as required.

Makes about 1 litre ($1^3/_4$ pints)   *Carbohydrate: none*

Cooked mayonnaise

5 egg yolks
1 tbsp cornflour
2 tbsp extra virgin oil
2 tbsp lemon juice
$^1/_2$ cup hot water
ground white pepper

In a small saucepan, combine the yolks with the cornflour, add the oil in a slow stream, whisking, and whisk in the lemon juice and hot water. Cook over a moderately low heat, whisking constantly, until thickened. Remove from the heat, season with salt and pepper, and transfer to a jar. Chill until cold.

Makes about 1 cup   *Carbohydrate: 7 grams*

Green Goddess dressing

1 garlic clove, halved
8 anchovy fillets, drained, reserving 1 tsp of the oil
1 minced spring onion
1 tsp minced fresh tarragon leaves
$^1/_2$ tbsp minced fresh parsley leaves
2 tsp minced fresh chives
2 tsp tarragon vinegar
1 cup mayonnaise

Rub a bowl with the cut garlic. In the bowl, mash the anchovies with the reserved oil, add the spring onion, tarragon, parsley, chives and vinegar and mayonnaise. Combine well. (At this stage the mixture will be very thick. It may be thinned with water to the desired consistency.)

The dressing may be used thick as a dip with prawns or vegetables, or thinned on salads or white fish.

Makes about 1$^1/_2$ cups   *Carbohydrate: negligible*

Chili dressing

1 tbsp double cream
3 tbsp mayonnaise
1 tbsp bottled chili sauce
2 tbsp finely chopped fresh parsley
1 small onion, finely chopped
1 tbsp finely chopped chives
pinch of cayenne pepper

Whip the cream until it just maintains soft peaks. Whisk the other ingredients in a bowl. Fold in the whipped cream gently but thoroughly.

Makes about 1 cup   *Carbohydrate: negligible*

Hard egg hollandaise

3 hard-boiled egg yolks
4 tsp lemon juice
100 g (4 oz) butter
finely chopped fresh herbs (if desired)

Blend the yolks in a food processor until smooth, add 2 tablespoons of boiling water and the lemon juice and blend the mixture until smooth and fluffy. In a small saucepan, heat the butter over a moderate heat until it begins to foam. With the food processor running, slowly pour in the butter in a thin stream and season to taste with the herbs, salt and white pepper.

Makes about 1 cup   *Carbohydrate: 1 gram*

Saffron garlic mayonnaise

$^1/_4$ tsp saffron threads
2 tsp lemon juice
275 ml ($^1/_2$ pint) mayonnaise
3 garlic cloves, crushed
pinch of cayenne pepper

Put the saffron on a saucer on a rack over a saucepan of boiling water and steam until brittle (3 or 4 minutes). Remove and crumble into a bowl. Whisk in the lemon juice, mayonnaise, garlic paste and cayenne pepper until the mixture is well combined.

Serve with fish soups, grilled seafood or chicken.

Makes about 1 cup   *Carbohydrate: 2 grams*

Oilless mayonnaise and dip

3 hard-boiled eggs
1 tbsp wine vinegar
3 tbsp plain yoghurt
2 tsp brown sugar or honey
small garlic clove
salt and pepper

Place all ingredients into a liquidiser and liquidise until
the mixture is smooth (about 3 minutes).

Makes about 1 cup   *Carbohydrate: negligible*

To make the oilless mayonnaise into a dip use a little less
yoghurt and add another egg. You can also add other
ingredients, such as anchovies, to make other flavours.

Desserts

Baked egg custard

3 large eggs
600 ml (1 pint) full-cream milk
$^1/_2$ tsp vanilla essence
6–8 drops liquid or granulated artificial sweetener
pinch of nutmeg

Break the eggs into an ovenproof dish and beat lightly. In a
small saucepan, heat the milk but do not allow to boil.
Add the sweetener and vanilla essence. Pour into the egg
mixture, stirring to ensure it is well mixed. Sprinkle with
nutmeg. Place the dish in a tray of water and bake in a

cool oven (150°C/300°F/Gas Mark 2) until the custard is just set (about 1 hour).

Serves 4   *Carbohydrate: 8 grams*

Apple snow

450 g (1 lb) cooking apples
2 egg whites
juice and zest of 1 lemon
liquid or granulated artificial sweetener

Make a shallow cut around the middle of each apple. Place them in a baking dish and bake in a moderate oven (180°C/350°F/Gas Mark 4) for 30 minutes. Remove the pulp from the apples and press it through a sieve. Add sweetener to taste and leave the mixture to cool. Meanwhile beat the egg whites until stiff. Add the apple mixture, a little at a time. Spoon into decorative dishes and chill well before serving.

Serves 4   *Carbohydrate: 10 grams*

Dark chocolate mousse with mandarin oranges

225 g (8 oz) continental dark chocolate (70% or more cocoa
    solids)
4 large eggs, separated
2 tbsp orange liqueur (or juice from mandarin oranges)
6 tbsp double cream
1 tin (295 g) mandarin oranges, drained

Line a shallow 200 mm (8 inch) round cake tin with clear film.
    Break up and melt the chocolate in a bowl over a pan of hot water. Beat the egg yolks and orange liqueur into the chocolate then fold in the cream, mixing well.
    In a separate bowl, whisk the egg whites until stiff, then gently fold them into the chocolate mixture.

Pour the mixture into the prepared cake tin, level the surface and chill in a refrigerator for several hours until set.

Turn out the mousse onto a plate and serve with the mandarin oranges.

Serves 6   *Carbohydrate: 11 grams*

Lemon soufflé

4 large eggs, separated
juice and zest of 1 lemon
3 tbsp caster sugar

Beat the egg yolks with the lemon and sugar until light and frothy. Whip the egg whites until stiff and fold into the lemon mixture. Pour into a buttered soufflé dish and bake in a hot oven (200°C/400°F/Gas Mark 6) for 10 minutes. This dish should be made as quickly as possible and served immediately.

Serves 4   *Carbohydrate: 12 grams*

Real vanilla ice-cream

4 large eggs
100 g (4 oz) caster sugar
400 ml (³/₄ pint) whipping cream
vanilla essence

Separate the eggs. In a bowl, whisk the egg whites until stiff. Add the yolks and sugar.

In another bowl, whip the cream until stiff. Combine the cream and the egg mixture and add the vanilla essence, then freeze.

Serves 4   *Carbohydrate: 25 grams*

Alternative ice-cream

Some very nice ice-cream can be made quickly and easily using just whipping cream and jam. Whip the cream until stiff and combine with lemon curd, black cherry jam, or any other smooth jam.

The next two recipes are quite high in carbohydrates but they contain no cereal starches. They are also quite rich so it is not likely that you could eat too much at one time!

Hazelnut cake

6 large eggs
130 g (5 oz) caster sugar
225 g (8 oz) ground hazelnuts
1 tbsp rum (or flavour to suit)

Grease one large loose-bottom sponge tin (9 inch) or two smaller.

Separate eggs. Add 2 tbsp of sugar to the yolks and beat until pale and foamy. Add hazelnuts and flavouring.

Whip egg whites with the remaining sugar until stiff. Fold in the hazelnut mixture.

Put into sponge tin and bake for approximately $1^1/_2$ hours at 120°C. (It is done when a wooden cocktail stick comes out cleanly when tested.)

Decorate with whipped cream and grated dark chocolate or cherries.

Serve with cream.

Serves 6   *Carbohydrate: 27 grams*

Chocolate cake (no-flour)

330 g (12 oz) dark continental chocolate (70% or more cocoa
   solids) broken into small pieces
5 whole eggs
140 g (5 oz) caster sugar
225 g (½ lb) unsalted butter, softened

Preheat oven to 160°C/325°F/Gas Mark 3.

Line a small loaf tin with greaseproof paper, grease and
flour it.

Beat the eggs with half the sugar until the volume
quadruples. This will take several minutes with an
electric mixer.

Heat the remaining sugar in a small pan with 125 ml
(4 fl oz) of water until the sugar has dissolved to a syrup.

Place the chocolate and butter in the hot syrup and stir
to combine. Remove from the heat and allow to cool
slightly.

Add the warm syrup to the eggs and continue to beat,
rather more gently, until completely combined – about 20
seconds, no more. Pour into the cake tin and place in a
bain marie of hot water. It is essential, if the cake is to
cook evenly, that the water comes level with the top of
the cake. Bake in the oven for 30 minutes or until set. Test
by placing the flat of your hand gently on the surface.

Leave to cool in the tin before turning out.

Serve with cream.

Serves 6   *Carbohydrate: 40 grams*

Most people love ice-cream but the commercial products
are suspect as far as their carbohydrate content – and
chemical content – is concerned. Fortunately, *real* ice-
cream is not only nicer, it is also healthier and less
fattening.

Strawberries and cream

Fresh strawberries and cream are delicious, and strawberries are low in carbohydrate. However, normally they are sugared, which increases the carbohydrate content considerably. If you think that you have to add sugar, try this: after washing the fruit, place for about 30 minutes in a pint of water in which a teaspoon of salt has been mixed, then drain and serve. You will be surprised how sweet they taste. The same can be done with raspberries, melon and apple.

Children's treats

Red fruit compôte

Choose a variety of mainly red, soft fruit: strawberries, raspberries, cherries, papaya, mango, melon, passion fruit, banana, pears, peach, and nectarines. Cut the large fruit into cubes or slices and mix all the fruit in a small amount of fresh orange juice. Marinate for an hour. Serve with unsweetened whipped cream.

Fruit jelly

300 ml (½ pint) orange juice
20 g (¾ oz) powdered gelatine
3 kiwi fruit, peeled sliced thinly
100 g (4 oz) washed strawberries, sliced in halves
½ a pink melon, sliced thinly
3 oranges, segmented
a few raspberries or strawberries

Heat half the orange juice in a small saucepan. Off the heat, sprinkle in the gelatine and stir well to dissolve. Reheat gently if any grains do not dissolve. Do not allow to boil. Add the rest of the juice, mix and set aside.

Using an empty butter wrapper, lightly grease a large loaf tin. Put the fruit into the tin in neat layers, kiwi fruit first. Scatter the raspberries throughout as you go.

When all the fruit is in, pour in the juice. Put in the fridge to set.

To turn out, run a blunt knife around the sides and warm the bottom. Place a serving plate on top and invert.

Serve with double cream or Greek yoghurt.

Fresh fruit trifle

This is a trifle based on the fruit jelly above.

1 pkt trifle sponges
fruit jelly (see above)
140 ml (½ pint) double cream
140 ml (½ pint) Greek yoghurt

Slice the sponges in half, lengthways, and place in the bottom of a serving bowl. Pour over the jelly and place in the fridge to set.

Whisk the cream until it is just firm and fold in the yoghurt. Spread this mixture over the jelly.

Decorate the top with the raspberries, or any other fruit except pineapple. But leave this until just before serving to avoid staining the cream.

Glossary

Amino-acids are the fundamental constituents of all proteins. There are twenty in the protein foods we eat and we need all of them. Our bodies can manufacture all but eight. These, called the *essential amino-acids*, must be obtained from protein in the diet. Not only must all eight be present, they should ideally be in these proportions:

one part tryptophan to
two parts each of phenylalanine and threonine to
three parts each of isoleucine, lysine, methionine and valine to
three and a half parts leucine.

You do not need to remember their names. When all are contained in a food, this is said to be complete protein. Egg whites contain all the essential amino-acids in the correct proportions. The best sources of the essential amino-acids, in approximately the right proportions, are foods such as liver, eggs, and dairy products. Soy beans are the only vegetable source of complete protein. Pulses, cereals and nuts all contain some but not all of the essential amino-acids and not in the required proportions. These are called incomplete proteins. Thus a vegetarian diet must contain a mixture of these for all eight essential amino-acids to be supplied.

Atheroma is degeneration of artery walls due to the formation of fatty plaques and scar tissue. Although atheroma narrows arteries and restricts blood flow, it is usually symptomless. However, it can cause complications in later life such as angina, heart attack, stroke and gangrene.

Bioavailability. The bioavailability of a nutrient in a foodstuff is a measure of the proportion of it which is absorbed into the bloodstream. Bioavailability is affected by a number of factors. For example, no enzyme in the human gut can digest the cellulose from which plant cell walls are made. Therefore, unless those walls are ruptured in some way, the nutrients inside a plant cell will not be available to the digestion. Cooking and chewing, which damage the cell walls, increase bioavailability. Phytic acid, which is found in bran, is an 'anti-nutrient'. This substance combines with a number of minerals to form a compound which is indigestible thus reducing their bioavailability.

Calorie. The calorie, or more correctly in dietary terms kilocalorie (kcal), is a unit of heat. It is the amount of heat required to raise the temperature of a kilogram of water by one degree Celsius.

Carbohydrates are one of the three main constituents of food. They are a large group of compounds which include sugars, starches, celluloses and gums. Apart from the indigestible starches (fibre), all carbohydrates are eventually broken down in the body into the simple sugar, glucose. Excess carbohydrate, not immediately needed by the body, is stored in the body: in the liver and muscles as glycogen, a form of starch and as fat. Glycogen is later broken down into glucose to be used as energy.

Cholesterol is a white waxy material. It is not a fat but a form of alcohol called a *lipid alcohol*. In higher animals, it is found in all cells and it is especially abundant in the brain and nervous tissue. In cells, it is used principally as a structural material – cell wall membranes are made of it. In these membranes, its ratio with other lipids has a large impact on the stability and permeability of the membranes. The myelin sheath which is the 'insulation' around nerves has the highest concentration of cholesterol. (Multiple sclerosis results from the breakdown of this myelin sheath.)

In addition to its structural function cholesterol performs other important functions: it is a precursor for several hormones, including both male and female sex hormones; in the liver it is used to make the bile acids and bile salts which are secreted into the gut as part of the digestive process; and it is used by the body to manufacture vitamin D in conjunction with sunlight.

Cholesterol and other substances in the blood are measured in milli-moles per litre (mmol/l) in Australia and Europe and in milligrams per decilitre (mg/dl) in the United States of America. Normal blood concentration of cholesterol is 3.6–7.8 mmol/l (140–300 mg/dl), but this rises naturally with age: at the age of fifty, for example, 9.0 mmol/l (346 mg/dl) would not be abnormal. The normal Western intake of cholesterol from food is 500–1,000 mg/day. However, the body uses considerably more than this and the extra required is synthesised from acetate mainly in the liver. Normally the amount of cholesterol in the blood from these two sources is constant because under feedback control, if more is eaten, the liver compensates by making less. On a low-cholesterol diet, the amount synthesised by the liver rises markedly.

Cholesterol is found in equal amounts in both the lean and fat portions of meat.

HDL and LDL Cholesterol. Cholesterol is transported around the body by a group of proteins combined with lipids called lipoproteins. The higher the ratio of proteins to lipids, the higher the density of the lipoprotein. Although one normally hears only of High Density Lipoprotein cholesterol (HDL, the 'good' cholesterol, which is believed by some to protect against heart disease) and Low Density Lipoprotein cholesterol (LDL, the 'bad' cholesterol, which is believed by some to cause heart disease), there are actually several distinct densities including Very Low Density (VLDL), and Intermediate Density; even HDL is split into HDL2 and HDL3.

Controls. When a medical trial is conducted it is usual to divide the people taking part in the trial into two groups. One group will be given the active treatment while the other will be given none. In this way doctors can assess the effectiveness of the treatment by measuring the differences between the two groups. The group that receives the treatment is called the 'intervention group' and the group that does not receive the treatment is known as the 'control group' or 'controls'.

Cro-Magnon. Our ancestors, whom we call Cro-Magnon, migrated into Europe from the Middle East around 35,000 years ago. They were fully modern men, identical in appearance to the modern European. They apparently had a culture all their own and made better weapons and tools than the Neanderthals. Like the Neanderthals, they occupied caves but in larger groups and on a more permanent basis.

Epidemiology is a branch of science which deals with diseases in population groups. It includes all forms of disease that relate to environmental and lifestyle factors.

Essential fatty acids (EFAs) are a group of three polyunsaturated fatty acids (once known as vitamin F) which the body needs but cannot synthesise itself. They are: arachidonic, linoleic and linolenic acid. Although all three are essential, the only one which need be included in the diet is linoleic acid, as the body can make the other two from it. Vegetable oils such as sunflower, safflower, soya and corn oils contain large quantities of linoleic acid. Animal fats also contain it but in smaller amounts. The body requires only small quantities of the essential fatty acids.

Fat is a substance which contains one or more fatty acids and is the principal form in which the body stores energy. It is also used as an insulating material, just beneath the skin and around some of the internal organs. Fat is essential in the diet to supply an adequate amount of essential fatty acids and for the absorption of the fat-soluble vitamins: A, D, E and K.

The chemical and physical properties of a fat are determined by the relative amounts of the various fatty acids of which it is composed. Generally, the more saturated the fatty-acid content, the harder the fat will be at room temperature; the more unsaturated its content, the runnier it will be.

Fatty acids. All fats are composed of fatty acids, of which there are dozens in nature. A fatty acid is an organic acid having long hydrocarbon chains with an even number of carbon molecules and a number of 'double bonds'. It is the difference between these that differentiates the various fatty acids. Some fatty acids can be synthesised in the body; the essential fatty acids cannot. Although there are many fatty acids, they are normally placed into one of two groups: saturated fatty acids or unsaturated fatty acids. *Saturated fatty acids* have no double bonds and this makes them stable. It also makes their hydrocarbon chain molecules straight and unbending, which in turn makes fats containing them hard at room temperature. The major saturated fatty acids are *palmitic acid* and *stearic acid*. *Unsaturated fatty acids* having one double bond are called *mono*unsaturated and those with two or more are *poly*unsaturated. The unsaturated fatty acids are not stable; they react gradually with oxygen in the air and become rancid. This oxygenation process produces molecules known as 'free radicals' which are known to have undesirable effects on the body. Oleic acid, a monounsaturated fatty acid, occurs in substantial quantities in all fats, especially in olive oil, where it forms seventy per cent of the fatty-acid content. Oleic acid is also the most abundant fatty acid in animal fats and in human fat. Linoleic acid, a polyunsaturated fatty acid with two double bonds, is the major fatty acid of vegetable seed oils such as sunflower, safflower, soya and corn oils, where it forms fifty-five to seventy per cent of their fatty-acid content. It is these which are used for the manufacture of 'high-in-polyunsaturates' margarines and as cooking oils. Human fats contain very little linoleic acid.

The fatty-acid content of some typical foods is tabled below. The total percentages are less than 100 because of the glycerol and other compounds that are present.

FATTY ACID CONTENT OF TYPICAL FOODS

	% fat	% of saturated fat	% mono-unsaturated fat	% poly-unsaturated fat
Milk – cow's	3.9	64	28	3
human	4.1	48	39	8
Cheese, Cheddar	33.5	63	27	4
Eggs	10.9	31	39	11
Beef	27.4	41	47	4
Pork	25.5	35	42	15
Chicken	12.8	30	45	20
Liver, lamb's	6.2	28	29	15
Mackerel	22.9	20	49	20
Butter	82.0	68	23	4
Margarine – hard	81.0	39	47	10
polyunsaturated	81.0	17	27	52
Blended cooking oil	99.9	13	25	58
Peanuts, roasted	49.0	12	38	37
Chocolate, milk	30.3	58	33	4

Fibre, or roughage as it used to be called, is that part of a plant which cannot be digested and absorbed in the human gut. Although, because of its indigestibility, it cannot be classed as a food, a certain amount of fibre is believed to be necessary for the correct functioning of the gut and the passage of materials through the intestines and bowel. Fibre falls into four groups: celluloses, of which plant cell walls are made; hemicelluloses; lignins, another constituent of cell walls which give a plant stiffness; and pectins. All fruits, vegetables and cereals contain fibre but the types of fibre differ in each.

The major fibre found in fruits is pectin. Not fibrous in texture, it has little effect on the faeces. The major fibre in vegetables is cellulose. In ruminant animals such as cows, cellulose is broken down and used as a food; in humans it passes straight through, as we have no enzymes to digest it. The sources of the greatest quantities of fibre are cereals, particularly bran and wholemeal flours. However, there is a penalty to pay. Cereal fibres are fundamentally different from vegetable and fruit fibre in that they also contain a material called phytate which binds with many nutrients, reduces their bioavailability and stops them from being digested.

Glucose is a simple sugar molecule. It is an important source of energy within the body. Glucose is the building block from which sugars and starches are composed. All sugar and starch carbohydrates are converted back to glucose by the process of digestion. Glucose is stored in the body's muscles in the form of glycogen. Any excess is converted and stored as fat.

Glycogen, a carbohydrate, is the principal form in which glucose is stored in the body, the counterpart of the starch that is stored in plants. It is stored in the liver and muscles, any excess being converted into and stored as fat. As glycogen it is readily broken down into glucose for use. After it has been converted into fat, however, the process is more difficult.

Intervention trials. Whenever a new drug, diet or other treatment is devised, it has to be tested to make sure that it is both effective and safe. In these circumstances the usual method is to select two groups of people who are matched for age, sex, lifestyle and so on. One, the *intervention* group, is then given the treatment while the other, the *control* group, is not. By comparing the responses of the two groups, it is possible to assess the efficacy and/or safety of the treatment.

To ensure that there is no bias and to minimise the placebo effect, where a medicine is tested, such intervention trials are usually 'double blind'. This means that neither the doctors administering the treatment nor the subjects taking part know who is receiving the active treatment and who is receiving an inactive placebo.

Ischaemic means 'lacking oxygen'. It usually refers to an inadequate flow of blood to a part of the body caused by constriction or blockage of the arteries supplying it.

Ketones are a group of organic compounds related to acetone. They are normal products formed during the metabolism of fats and can be used by the body as a source of energy. Elevated levels arise when there is an imbalance in fat metabolism, as may occur in diabetes or starvation.

Lipids are a group of naturally occurring compounds which are soluble in solvents such as alcohol but not in water. The group includes fats and steroids that are important constituents of our diet, not only because of their high energy value but because they are associated with certain vitamins and essential fatty acids.

Metabolism is the sum of all the chemical and physical processes which take place within the living body to enable its continued growth and function. It is also the process whereby energy and heat are made available to the body. The *Basal Metabolic Rate* (BMR) is the minimum amount of energy the body needs to expend to maintain vital processes such as breathing, circulation, hormone production and digestion.

Phytate (or phytic acid) is a compound found in certain foods that binds with minerals such as calcium, iron and zinc to form indigestible compounds which the body treats as waste products. Foods high in phytates therefore inhibit the absorption of these minerals, leading to deficiencies. Whole-grain cereals, soy beans and peanuts are the major sources of phytate.

Proteins are essential components in the body, being the materials from which the organs, muscles and tissues are made. Organic compounds composed of hydrogen, carbon, oxygen and nitrogen, they are synthesised in the body from amino-acids, which in turn are absorbed from digested dietary proteins.

Protein is unstable. Body cells undergo a constant cycle of breakdown and rebuilding. Amino-acids in the cells have to be replaced on a daily basis, and newly digested amino-acids in food are used for this purpose, so your daily intake of proteins must always be sufficient. Inadequate protein intake will lead to deficiency diseases. Any excess can be used to supply energy.

Triglycerides are the form in which fat is stored in the body. They are lipids composed of glycerol combined with three fatty acids, and are synthesised in the body from the digestion of dietary fat. They are transported around the body with Very Low Density (VLDL) cholesterol.

Appendix

Carbohydrate content and Glycaemic Index of common foods

Carbohydrate content of common foods

For easy reference, below is a list of the carbohydrate content (in grams) of common foods in normal servings. As all foods from animals, fish and birds are low in carbohydrate and may be eaten freely, these are not included. Only foods of vegetable origin, and then only those which have a relatively concentrated carbohydrate content, need be avoided.

The glycaemic index

The glycaemic index is a relatively new measure of a food's ability to raise blood sugar and insulin levels and, thus, it is a good gauge of the relative amount of fat your body will pack away in your fat cells. The index was developed in 1981 to help diabetics determine what foods they could safely eat, but it has also proved very useful in the treatment of obesity. The glycaemic index is a numerical indication of how much your blood sugar rises over a period of two to three hours after eating. The higher the number, the faster a food raises blood sugar levels.

When the glycaemic index was first developed, scientists believed that simple sugars were digested more quickly than complex carbohydrates and raised blood sugar levels quickly. This was why diabetics were advised to cut down on sweets and eat more 'complex carbohydrates', i.e. starches such as those found in bread and pasta. We now know, however, that these complex starches are also digested quickly and have a major effect on blood sugar levels. As the glycaemic indices of foods have been determined there have been some notable surprises. A baked potato, for example, is a greater offender than table sugar. The grains wheat, barley, rice, and oats tend to have high glycaemic indices, yet that for pearl barley is very low.

About 300 foods have been tested. Most are high-carbohydrate foods for the simple reason that it is carbohydrates that are the problem; proteins and fats have little effect on blood sugar levels and are safe for diabetics and the overweight to eat.

The glycaemic index also depends on other factors such as how ripe fruits are, whether they are cooked or raw and even on variety and method of processing. In underripe bananas, the carbohydrate content is largely starch. As the banana ripens this turns to sugar. The glycaemic index of underripe bananas is 43; for ripe bananas it is nearly double at 74. Not surprisingly, perhaps, particle size also has a marked effect on how quickly a carbohydrate is digested and raises blood sugar levels. In tests on wheat, maize and oats, whole grains had the lowest glycaemic index number. As the grains were ground into progressively finer flour, through cracked grains, coarse flour to fine flour, so their glycaemic indices progressively rose.

The way to use glycaemic indices is to be increasingly wary as the numbers get higher. Anything with a number over about 50 should be reduced and those foods whose glycaemic index is over about 80 should be avoided altogether, at least while you are actively trying to lose weight.

A list of foods and their glycaemic index appears below. You will notice that cereals and sugary foods tend to have the highest glycaemic index, which is as you would expect, although there are some notable exceptions and some surprises.

Food	Carbohydrate (grams)	Food	Carbohydrate (grams)

Fruit

Food	Carbohydrate (grams)	Food	Carbohydrate (grams)
Apple, small	10	juice, unsweetened, 275 ml (½ pint)	20
medium	13	Grapes, 25 g (1 oz)	4
large	21	Melon, raw, 175 g (6 oz)	5
Apricot, raw	2	Nectarine, raw, 150 g (5 oz)	16
dried	10	Orange, medium	9
Banana, ripe, small	15	Orange juice, 275 ml (½ pint)	24
medium	16	Peach, medium	9
Blackberries, raw, 25 g (1 oz)	2	Pear, medium	14
Cherries, raw, 25 g (1 oz))	40	Pineapple, raw, 25 g (1 oz)	3
Clementine	5	Plums, raw, 110 g (4 oz)	10
Currants, dried, 25 g (1 oz)	18	Prunes, dried, with stones	9
Damsons, raw, 25 g (1 oz)	2	Raspberries, raw, 25 g (1 oz)	2
Dates, dried, 25 g (1 oz)	18	Rhubarb, stewed, no sugar, 150 g (5 oz)	1
Fig, raw, one	4	Strawberries, raw, 25 g (1 oz)	2
Gooseberries, raw, 25 g (1 oz)	1		
Grapefruit, raw, 200 g (7 oz)	5		

Nuts

Food	Carbohydrate (grams)	Food	Carbohydrate (grams)
Almonds, 25 g (1 oz)	1	Cobs, 25 g (1 oz)	2
Brazils, 25 g (1 oz)	1	Coconut, raw, 25 g (1 oz)	1
Cashews, roasted, 110 g (4 oz)	18	Coconut, desiccated, 25 g (1 oz)	2
Chestnuts, shelled, 25 g (1 oz)	10	Hazelnuts, 25 g (1 oz)	2

Food	Carbohydrate (grams)	Food	Carbohydrate (grams)
Cereals			
Butter biscuits, 2	15	Pasta (all types), dry, 25 g (1 oz)	7
Cream crackers, 4	19	Pasta verde, dry, 25 g (1 oz)	22
Digestive biscuits, 2	19	cooked, 25 g (1 oz)	6
Water biscuits, 4	21	Pastry, 25 g (1 oz)	10–14
Bread, small slice	12	Porridge, made with water, 110 g (4 oz)	9
Croissant	30		
Crumpet	16	Rice, white, raw, 25 g (1 oz)	25
Muffin	28	boiled, 25 g (1 oz)	8
Roll	30		
Flour, plain, 25 g (1 oz)	23	Sugar, 25 g (1 oz)	28
Oats, raw, 25 g (1 oz)	21	Honey, 25 g (1 oz)	22

The carbohydrate content of breakfast cereals is marked on the packet.

Vegetables

Most green vegetables are low in carbohydrate and are therefore not listed. It is the root vegetables and seeds which tend to have a relatively high carbohydrate content. They are listed below. As a rough guide, restrict yourself to about a cup of vegetables (measured after cooking) per meal. Greens may be eaten in larger quantities.

Food	Carbohydrate (grams)	Food	Carbohydrate (grams)
Beans, baked, 2 tbs	4	Lentils, dried, 25 g (1 oz)	15
broad, raw, 25 g (1 oz)	2	Onion, medium	3
butter, dried, 25 g (1 oz)	14	Parsnips, raw, 25 g (1 oz)	3
French, raw, 25 g (1 oz)	0	Peas, raw, 25 g (1 oz)	3
haricot, dried, 25 g (1 oz)	13	Potatoes, raw, 110 g (4 oz)	24
runner, raw, 25 g (1 oz)	1		
Beetroot, raw, medium	6	Sweetcorn, canned, 25 g (1 oz)	5
Carrots, raw, 110 g (4 oz)	5	Turnips, raw, 25 g (1 oz)	1
Corn on the cob, raw, medium	34		

Carbohydrate content of foods and their glycaemic index (GI)

This table gives the carbohydrate content of a wider range of foods in grams per 100 grams (3¹/₂ oz) and their glycaemic index (GI) where it is known. Where no glycaemic index rating is given, this is because it hasn't yet been determined. In the cases where the food is largely or wholly animal-based, the glycaemic index would be irrelevant.

Food	Carbohydrate (grams per 100 g)	GI	Food	Carbohydrate (grams per 100 g)	GI
Milk					
Cream, single	3		liquid, skimmed	5	46
Milk, liquid, whole	5	39	dried, skimmed	50	46
			Yoghurt, low-fat, natural	10	20
			low-fat, fruit	18	47
Cheese					
Cheddar	0		Feta	0	
Cottage	1		Brie	0	
Cheese spread	1				
Meat					
Bacon, rashers	0		Liver, lamb's, fried	0	
Beef, mince, stewed	0		Luncheon meat	3	
stewing steak	0		Pâté, average	1	
Black pudding, fried	15		Pork chop, cooked	0	
Chicken, roast, meat and skin	0		Sausage, beef, cooked	15	40
Corned beef	0		pork, cooked	11	40
Ham	0		Steak and kidney pie	22	
Kidney, pig's, fried	0		Turkey, roast, meat and skin	0	
Lamb, roast	0				

Food	Carbohydrate (grams per 100 g)	GI	Food	Carbohydrate (grams per 100 g)	GI

Fish

Food	Carbohydrate	GI	Food	Carbohydrate	GI
White fish	0		Pilchards, canned in tomato sauce	1	
Cod, fried	7		Prawns, boiled	0	
Fish fingers	16	54	Sardines, canned in oil, fish only	0	
Herrings	0		Tuna in oil	0	
Mackerel	0				

Eggs

Eggs, boiled or fried	0	

Fats

Food	Carbohydrate	Food	Carbohydrate
Lard, cooking fat, dripping	0	Margarine, average	0
		Cooking and salad oil	0

Preserves, etc.

Food	Carbohydrate	GI	Food	Carbohydrate	GI
Chocolate, milk	59	70	Sugar, white	105	92
Honey	76	83	Syrup	79	
Jam	69		Peppermints	100	
Marmalade	70				

Vegetables

Food	Carbohydrate	GI	Food	Carbohydrate	GI
Aubergines	3		Courgettes, raw	5	
Baked beans	15	69	Cucumber	2	
Beans, runner, boiled	3		Lentils, cooked	17	41
Beans, red kidney, raw	45	42	Lettuce	1	
Beans, soya, boiled	9	25	Mushrooms	0	
Beetroot, boiled	10	91	Onion	5	
Brussels sprouts, boiled	2		Parsnips, cooked	14	139
Cabbage, raw	3		Peas, frozen, boiled	11	68
boiled	2		Peas canned, processed	19	
Carrots, old	5	101	Peppers, green	2	
Cauliflower, cooked	1		Potatoes, boiled	18	87
Celery	1				

Food Carbohydrate (grams per 100 g)		GI	Food Carbohydrate (grams per 100 g)		GI

Vegetables (contd)

Food	Carbohydrate	GI	Food	Carbohydrate	GI
Potatoes, fried (chips)	34	107	Sweet potato	22	77
oven chips	30		Tomatoes, fresh	3	
roast	26		Turnips, cooked	2	
Potato crisps	50	77	Watercress	1	
Spinach, boiled	1		Yam, boiled	30	73
Sweetcorn, canned	17	78			

Fruit

Food	Carbohydrate	GI	Food	Carbohydrate	GI
Apples	12	54	Lemon juice	2	
Apricots, canned			Mango	15	80
in syrup	28	91	Melon, cantaloupe, raw	4	93
stewed, no sugar	5		Mulberries, raw	7	
dried	43	44	Nectarine, raw	10	
Avocado pear	2		Oranges	9	63
Bananas, ripe	19	77	Orange juice	9	74
Blackberries, raw	7		Peaches	9	60
Blackcurrants	7		canned in syrup	23	67
Cherries	12	32	Pears	11	53
Clementine	8		Pineapple	12	94
Cranberries, raw	4		Plums	8	55
Currants, dried	59		Prunes, dried	40	
Dates, dried	64		Raisins	60	91
Figs, dried	53		Raspberries	6	
Gooseberries, raw	4		Rhubarb, cooked,		
cooked, unsweetened	3		no sugar	1	
Grapes	16	66	Strawberries	6	
Grapefruit	5	36	Sultanas	65	80

Food	Carbohydrate (grams per 100 g)	GI	Food	Carbohydrate (grams per 100 g)	GI

Nuts

Food	Carbohydrate	GI	Food	Carbohydrate	GI
Almonds	4		Hazelnuts	7	
Brazils	4		Peanuts, roasted, salted	9	21
Cashews	27		Peanut butter	13	
Coconut, desiccated	6		Walnuts	3	

Cereals

Food	Carbohydrate	GI	Food	Carbohydrate	GI
Biscuits, chocolate	67		Flour, white	77	77
plain, digestive	69	84	wholemeal	63	
semi-sweet	75	79	Pearl barley	79	20
Bread, brown	44		Popcorn	66	79
white	49	101	Rice, raw	86	
wholemeal	42	99	instant, boiled 6 mins	128	
Chelsea bun	58		Spaghetti, raw	74	59
Cream crackers	68	102	Tapioca	90	115
Crispbread, rye	71	93			

Breakfast cereals

Food	Carbohydrate	GI	Food	Carbohydrate	GI
Cornflakes	85	119	Oats, porridge	66	87
Muesli	66	80	Weetabix	70	100

Cakes and pastries

Food	Carbohydrate	GI	Food	Carbohydrate	GI
Chocolate cake with butter icing	53		Jam tarts	63	
Fruit cake, rich	51		Plain cake, Madeira	58	

Puddings

Food	Carbohydrate	GI	Food	Carbohydrate	GI
Apple pie	57		Custard	17	61
Bread and butter pudding	17		Ice-cream, dairy	21	87
Cheesecake, frozen, fruit topping	33		Rice pudding	20	
			Trifle	20	

Beverages

Food	Carbohydrate	GI	Food	Carbohydrate	GI
Chocolate, drinking	77	49	Fanta	97	
Cocoa powder	12		Lucozade	136	

NOTE: Alcohol. There is some dispute over the effect of alcohol on the metabolism. One theory has it that alcohol reduces the combustion of fat in the body in a similar way to carbohydrate. On the other hand, Banting drank up to six glasses of claret each day and a glass of rum most evenings – and still lost weight. By dilating the blood vessels in the skin, making it work harder, alcohol may step up the metabolism sufficiently to compensate for the added calories taken in the alcohol. There is also experimental evidence that such increased metabolism coupled with increased loss of water from the skin and in urine could result in weight loss. Alcohol does not raise blood sugar or insulin levels.

Bibliography

In medical journals, a note of each reference is made with the point it is making in the discussion. As this can tend to distract the reader, these notes have been omitted from this book. However, I believe that the reader should have the opportunity of checking the references. For this reason they are listed below in the order in which they are used.

Large teaching hospitals have medical libraries to which members of the public may gain access if permission is sought. Journals are usually stored in alphabetical and date order. There is an *Index Medicus* for each year which indexes all reports, papers, studies, letters, and so on by subject and by author.

Reference formats vary from journal to journal. Those below all follow a standard pattern for ease of use. The format used is: Author, title, *journal*, year, volume, (part), first page of article.

Introduction
Wooley S C, Garner D M. Dietary treatments for obesity are ineffective. *Br Med J.* 1994; 309: 655.

Garrow J S. Should obesity be treated? *Br Med J.* 1994; 309: 654.

Hirsch J. Herman award lecture, 1994: Establishing a biologic basis for obesity. *Am J Clin Nutr.* 1994; 60: 613.

Grace C, Summerbell C, Kopelman P. An audit of dietary treatment modalities and weight loss outcomes in a specialist obesity clinic. *J Human Nutr Diet.* 1998; 11: 197.

Chapter 1: The High-Fat Diet Debate

Banting W. *Letter on Corpulence to the Public.* 1863.

Densmore H. *How to Reduce Fat.* H Densmore, Los Angeles. 1895.

Stefansson V. *The Fat of The Land.* Macmillan & Co. New York. 1956.

Change your diet: eat like an Eskimo. *Daily Mail.* 8 June 1999; 42.

Lyon D M, Dunlop D M. The treatment of obesity: a comparison of the effects of diet and of thyroid extract. *Quart J Med.* 1932; 1: 331.

Kekwick A, Pawan G L S. Calorie intake in relation to body-weight changes in the obese. *Lancet.* 1956; ii: 155.

Hausberger F X, Milstein S W. Dietary effect on lipogenesis in adipose tissue. *J Bio Chem.* 1955; 214: 483.

Kekwick A. The metabolism of fat. *J R Coll Gen Pract.* 1967; 13 (Suppl 7): 95.

National Advisory Committee on Nutrition Education. *A Discussion Paper on Proposals for Nutritional Guidelines for Health Education in Britain.* HEC. 1983.

Committee on Medical Aspects of Food Policy. *Diet and Cardiovascular Disease.* DHSS. 1984.

Pennington A W. Pyruvic acid metabolism in obesity. *Am J Dig Dis.* February 1955; 33.

Chapter 2: It's In Our Genes

Lee R B. *What hunters do for a living, or how to make out on scarce resources.* In R B Lee, I DeVore, eds. *Man The Hunter.* Aldine, Chicago. 1968.

— *The !Kung San: men, women and work in a foraging society.* Cambridge University Press, New York. 1979.

Gaulin S J C, Konner M. *On the natural diet of primates, including humans.* In: Wurtman R Y, Wurtman J J, eds. *Nutrition and The Brain.* Vol 1, Raven Press, New York. 1977.

Bryant V M, Williams-Dean G. The Coprolites of Man. *Scientific American.* January 1975.

Crawford M, Crawford S. *The Food We Eat Today.* Spearman, London. 1972.

Leopold A C. Toxic Substances in Plants and Food Habits of Early Man. *Science.* 1972.

Hawkes J G. *The Hunting Hypothesis.* In: Ardrey R, ed. *The Hunting Hypothesis.* Collins, London. 1976.

Yudkin J. *Archaeology and the nutritionist.* In: Ardrey R, ed. *The Hunting Hypothesis.* Collins, London. 1976.

Cleave T L. The neglect of natural principles in current medical practice. *J RN Med Serv.* 1956; XLII, No 2: 55.

McGregor-Robertson J. *The Household Physician. Vol 2.* The Gresham Publishing Co. Ltd. London.

Given H D C. *A New Angle on Health.* John Bale, Sons & Danielsson Ltd. 1935.

McClellan W S, Du Bois E F. Prolonged meat diets with a study of kidney function and ketosis. *J Biol Chem*. 1930; 87: 651.

Orr J B, Gilks J L. *Studies of Nutrition: The Physique and Health of Two African Tribes*. HMSO. London. 1931.

McCormick J, Elmore-Meegan M. Maasai Diet. *Lancet*. 1992; 340: 1042.

Sandler B P. *How to Prevent Heart Attacks*. Lee Foundation for Nutritional Research, Milwaukee, Wisconsin.

Rifkind B M, *et al*. Effects of short-term sucrose restriction on serum-lipid levels. *Lancet*. 24 December 1961.

Yudkin J. Dietary sucrose and the behaviour of blood platelets. *Proc Nutr Soc*.1969; 29.

Flint F J. The factor of infection in heart failure. *Br Med J*. 1954; 2: 1018.

How important are respiratory infections as a cause of heart failure? *Arteriosclerosis*. 7 September, 1955.

Makinen K K. The role of sucrose and other sugars in the development of dental caries: A review. *Int Dent J*. 1972; 22 (3): 363.

Cleave T L. *The Saccharine Disease*. Keats Publishing, New Canaan, Conn. 1975.

Ahrens R A. Sucrose, hypertension and heart disease: A historical perspective. *Am J Clin Nutr*. 1974; 27.

Chapter 3: Eat Less, Weigh More!

Rose G A, Williams R T. Metabolic studies on large eaters and small eaters. *Br J Nutr*. 1961; 15: 188.

Shimomura Y, *et al*. Opiate receptors, food intake and obesity. *Physiology and Behaviour*. 1982; 28: 441.

Prentice A M, Jebb S A, Black A E. Extrinsic sugar as a vehicle for dietary fat. *Lancet*. 1995; 346: 695.

Jenkins D A J, *et al*. Glycemic index of foods: a physiological basis for carbohydrate exchange. *Am J Clin Nutr*. 1981; 34: 362.

Heaton K W, *et al*. Particle size of wheat, maize and oat test meals: effect on plasma glucose and insulin responses and on the rate of starch digestion in vitro. *Am J Clin Nutr*. 1988; 47: 675.

Miller J B. International tables of glycemic index. *Am J Clin Nutr*. 1995; 62 (Suppl): 871S.

Jung R T, *et al*. Reduced thermogenesis in obesity. *Nature*. 1979; 279: 323.

Himms-Hagen J. Obesity may be due to a malfunctioning of brown fat. *Can Med Assn J*. 1979; 121: 1361.

— *Thyroid hormones and thermogenesis*. In L Girardier, N J Stock, eds. *Mammalian Thermogenesis*, Chapman and Hall, London. 1983.

Rothwell N J, Stock N J. A role for brown adipose tissue in diet-induced thermogenesis. *Nature*. 1979; 281: 31.

Schutz Y, *et al*. Diet-induced thermogenesis measured over a whole day in obese and non-obese women. *Am J Clin Nutr*. 1984; 40: 542.

Chapter 4: The Cholesterol Myth

Gofman J W, *et al.* The role of lipids and lipoproteins in atherosclerosis. *Science.* 1950; 111: 166.

Strong J P, McGill H C jr. The natural history of coronary atherosclerosis. *Am J Pathol.* 1962; 40: 37.

Enos W F, Holmes R H, Beyer J. Coronary disease among United States soldiers killed in action in Korea. Preliminary report. *JAMA.*1953; 152: 1090.

Keys A. Atherosclerosis: a problem in newer public health. *J Mt Sinai Hosp.* 1953; 20: 118.

McMichael J M. Fats and atheroma: an inquest. *Br Med J.* 1979; 279: 890.

— Diet and coronary disease. *Acta Med Scand.* 1980; 207(3): 151.

Smith E B, Smith R H. Early changes in aortic intima. *Atheroscler Rev.* 1976; I: 119.

Wass V J, *et al.* Does the nephrotic syndrome increase the risk of cardiovascular disease? *Lancet.* 1979; ii: 664.

Moore R A. Variation in serum cholesterol. *Lancet.* 1988; ii: 682.

Editorial. Virus infections and atherosclerosis. *Lancet.* 1978; ii: 821.

Houghton J L, von Dohlen T W, Frank M J. Myocardial ischaemia without atherosclerosis. *Postgrad Med.* 1989; 86 (5): 121.

Woodhill J M, *et al. Low fat, low cholesterol diet in secondary prevention of coronary heart disease.* In D Kritschevky, R Paoletti, W L Holmes, eds. *Drugs, lipid metabolism and atherosclerosis.* New York: Plenum Press. 1978: 317.

Diet and Cardiovascular Disease. Committee on Medical Aspects of Food Policy. DHSS. 1984.

Kannel W B, Gordon T. *The Framingham Diet Study: diet and the regulations of serum cholesterol (Sect 24).* Washington DC, Dept of Health, Education and Welfare. 1970.

Kannel W B, Castelli W P. Is serum cholesterol an anachronism? *Lancet.* 1979; 2: 950.

Multiple Risk Factor Intervention Trial. *JAMA.* 1982; 248: 1465.

Nichols A B, *et al.* Daily nutritional intake and serum lipid levels: The Tecumseh Study. *Am J Clin Nutr.* 1976; 29: 1384.

World Health Organisation. European Collaborative Group. Multi-factorial trial in the prevention of coronary heart disease: 3. Incidence and mortality results. *Eur Heart J.* 1983; 4: 141.

Salonen J T, *et al.* Changes in morbidity and mortality during comprehensive community programme to control cardiovascular diseases during 1972-1977 in North Karelia. *Br Med J.* 1979; iv: 1178.

Puska P. The North Karelia Project: a community based programme for the prevention of heart and vascular disease. *Duodecim* (Helsinki). 1985; 101(23): 2281.

Lipid Research Clinic Programme. LRC-CPPT results. Reduction in incidence of coronary heart disease. *JAMA*. 1984; 251: 351.

Ravnskov V. Cholesterol lowering trials in coronary heart disease: frequency of citation and outcome. *Br Med J*. 1992; 305: 15.

Strandberg T E, Salomaa V V, Naukkarinen V A, *et al*. Long term mortality after 5-year multifactorial primary prevention of cardiovascular diseases in middle-aged men. *JAMA*. 1991; 266: 1225.

Gortner W A. Nutrition in the United States, 1900 to 1974. *Cancer Res*. 1975; 35: 3246.

Barker D J P, Osmond C. Diet and coronary heart disease in England and Wales during and after the second world war. *J Epidemiol Com Hlth*. 1986; 40: 37.

McKeigne P M, Miller G P, Marmot M G. Coronary heart disease in South Asians overseas: A review. *J Clin Epidemiol*. 1989; 42(7): 597.

Marmot M G. Interpretation of Trends in Coronary Heart Disease Mortality. *Acta Med Scand*. 1985 (Suppl); 701: 58.

Beaglehole R, *et al*. Cholesterol and mortality in New Zealand Maoris. *Br Med J*. 1980; 1: 285.

Ahrens E H. Dietary fats and coronary heart disease: unfinished business. *Lancet*. 1979; 2: 1345.

Dedichen J. Cholesterol and arteriosclerosis again. Are we on the wrong track? *Tidsskr Nor Laegeforen*. 1976; 96: 915-9.

Pearce M L, Dayton S. Incidence of cancer in men on a diet high in polyunsaturated fat. *Lancet*. 1971; 1: 464.

Hofmann A F, Northfield T C, Thistle J L. Can a cholesterol-lowering diet cause gallstones? *New Eng J Med*. 1973; 288 (1): 46.

Willett W C, *et al*. Intake of trans fatty acids and risk of coronary heart disease among women. *Lancet*. 1993; 341: 581.

Carroll K K. Dietary fats and cancer. *Am J Clin Nutr*. 1991; 53: 1064S.

France T, Brown P. Test-tube cancers raise doubts over fats. *New Scientist*, 7 December 1991, p 12.

Kearney R. Promotion and prevention of tumour growth – effects of endotoxin, inflammation and dietary lipids. *Int Clin Nutr Rev*. 1987; 7: 157.

Uldall P R, *et al*. *Lancet* 1974; ii: 514.

Balter M. Europe: as many cancers as cuisines. *Science*. 1991; 254: 114.

DesBordes C, Lea M A. Effects of C18 fatty acid isomers on DNA synthesis in hepatoma and breast cancer cells. *Anticancer-Res*. 1995; 15: 2017-21.

Koh H K. Cutaneous melanoma. *N Eng J Med*. 1991; 325: 171.

MacKie R, Hunter J A A, *et al*. Cutaneous malignant melanoma, Scotland, 1979-89. *Lancet*. 1992; 339: 971.

Takematsu H, *et al*. *Melanoma in Japan: experience at Tohoku University Hospital Sendai*. In C M Balch, G W Milton, eds. *Cutaneous Melanoma*. Philadelphia: Lippincott. 1984: 499.

Wolk A, *et al.* A Prospective Study of Association of Monounsaturated Fat and Other Types of Fat With Risk of Breast Cancer. *Arch Intern Med.* 1998;158: 41-45.

Ip C, Scimeca J A, Thompson H. Effect of timing and duration of dietary conjugated linoleic acid on mammary cancer prevention. *Nutr Cancer.* 1995; 24: 241.

Rose G A, *et al.* Corn oil in treatment of ischaemic heart disease. *Br Med J.* 1965; 1: 1531.

Fractured neck of femur: prevention and management. A report of the Royal College of Physicians, London. 1989.

Editorial: Why so many fractured hips? *Lancet.* 1989; 1: 57.

Fehily A M. Dietary determinants of bone mass and fracture risk: a review. *J Hum Nutr and Diet.* 1989; 2: 299.

Wargovich M J, Baer A R. Basic and Clinical Investigations of Dietary Calcium in the Prevention of Colorectal Cancer. *Prev Med.* 1989; 18: 672.

BBC. Horizon: The Poison That Waits. BBC2 broadcast 16 January 1989.

Bishop N, McGraw M, Ward N. Aluminium in infant formulas. *Lancet.* 1989; i: 490.

Golden B E, Golden M H N. Plasma zinc, rate of weight gain and the energy cost of tissue deposition in children recovering from malnutrition on cows' milk or a soya protein based diet. *Am J Clin Nutr.* 1981; 34: 892.

Prasad A. The role of zinc in gastrointestinal and liver disease. *Clin Gastroenterol.* 1983; 12: 713.

Aggett P, Davies N. Some nutritional aspects of trace elements. *J Inter Metab Dis.* 1983; 6(2): 22.

Hambidge M. The role of zinc and other trace metals in paediatric nutrition and health. *Paediat Clin N Am.* 1977; 24: 95.

Bryce-Smith D, Simpson R. Anorexia, depression and zinc deficiency. *Lancet.* 1984; ii: 1162.

Fonesca V, Harvard C. Electrolyte disturbances and cardiac failure with hypomagnesaemia in anorexia nervosa. *Br Med J.* 1985; 291: 1680.

Meadows N, *et al.* Zinc and small babies. *Lancet.* 1981; ii: 1135.

Bryce-Smith D. Environmental chemical influences on behaviour and mentation. John Jeyes lecture. *Chem Soc Rev.* 1986; 15: 93.

McMichael A, *et al.* A prospective study of serial maternal zinc levels and pregnancy outcome. *Early Human Development.* 1982 (Elsevier); 7: 59.

Addy D. Happiness is: iron. *Br Med J.* 1986; 292: 969.

Luk'ianova E M. Diagnosis of vitamin D deficiency rickets. *Pediatriia.* 1988; (3): 15.

Adelman R. Nutritional rickets. *Am J Dis Child.* 1988; 142(4): 414.

Clements M R. The problem of rickets in UK Asians. *J Hum Nutr Diet.* 1989; 2: 105.

Hughes R E. A new look at dietary fibre. *Hum Nutr Clin Nutr.* 1986; 40c: 81.

Hughes R E, Johns E. Apparent relation between dietary fibre and reproductive function in the female. *Ann Hum Biol.* 1985; 12: 325.

Lloyd T, *et al.* Inter-relationships of diet, athletic activity, menstrual status and bone density in collegiate women. *Am J Clin Nutr.* 1987; 46: 681.

Southgate D A T. Minerals, trace elements and potential hazards. *Am J Clin Nutr.* 1987; 45: 1256.

Wasan H S, Goodlad R A. Fiber-supplemented foods may damage your health. *Lancet.* 1996; 348: 319-20.

Yusuf S, Furberg C D. *Single factor trials: control through lifestyle changes.* In A G Olsson, ed. *Atherosclerosis.* Edinburgh: Churchill-Livingstone. 1987: 389.

Davey Smith G, Song F, Sheldon T A. Cholesterol lowering and mortality: the importance of considering initial level of risk. *Br Med J.* 1993; 306: 1367.

McMichael A J, *et al.* Dietary and endogenous cholesterol and human cancer. *Epidemiol Rev.* 1984; 6: 192.

Cambien F, *et al.* Total serum cholesterol and cancer mortality in a middle aged male population. *Am J Epid.* 1980; 112: 388.

Garcia-Palmieri M R, *et al.* An apparent inverse relationship between serum cholesterol and cancer mortality in Puerto Rico. *Am J Epid.* 1981; 114: 29.

Kozarevic D, *et al.* Serum cholesterol and mortality: the Yugoslavian cardiovascular diseases study. *Am J Epid.* 1981; 114: 21.

Hiatt R A, Fireman B H. Serum cholesterol and the incidence of cancer in a large cohort. *J Chronic Dis.* 1986; 39: 861.

Schatzkin A, *et al.* Serum cholesterol and cancer in the NHANES I epidemiologic follow up study. *Lancet.* 1987; ii: 298.

Kagan A, *et al.* Serum cholesterol and mortality in a Japanese-American population: the Honolulu heart program. *Am J Epid.* 1981; 114: 11.

Isles C G, *et al.* Plasma cholesterol, coronary heart disease and cancer in the Renfrew and Paisley survey. *Br Med J.* 1989; 298: 920.

Winawer S J, *et al.* Declining Serum Cholesterol Levels Prior to Diagnosis of Colon Cancer. *JAMA.* 1990; 263 (15): 2083.

Shimamoto T, *et al.* Trends for Coronary Heart Disease and Stroke and Their Risk Factors in Japan. *Circulation.* 1989; 3: 503.

Cholesterol in the prediction of atherosclerotic disease: new perspectives based on the Framingham Study. *Ann Int Med.* 1979; 90: 85-91.

Gillman M W, *et al.* Inverse association of dietary fat with development of ischemic stroke in men. *JAMA.* 1997; 278: 2145.

Corrigan F M, *et al.* Dietary supplementation with zinc sulphate, sodium selenite and fatty acids in early dementia of Alzheimer's Type II: Effects on lipids. *J Nutr Med.* 1991; 2: 265-71.

Foreman J. Cholesterol curb urged for children over 2. *The Boston Globe.* 9 April 1991: 1, 4.

Child mortality under age 5 per 1,000. in *Britannia Book of the Year 1992.* Encyclopaedia Britannica, Chicago.

Weverling-Rijnsburger A W E, *et al.* Total cholesterol and risk of mortality in the oldest old. *Lancet.* 1997; 350: 1119.

Jonsson A, Sigvaldason H, Sigfusson N. Total cholesterol and mortality after age 80 years. *Lancet.* 1997; 350: 1778.

Hulley S, *et al.* Editorial on Conference on low blood cholesterol. *Circulation.* 1992; 86 (3): 1026-9.

Report on the US National Heart, Lung and Blood Institute Conference on low blood cholesterol: Mortality associations. *Circulation* 1992; 86 (3): 1046-60.

Oliver M F. Reducing Cholesterol Does Not Reduce Mortality. *JACC.* 1988; 12(3): 814.

McCormick J, Skrabanek P. Coronary heart disease is not preventable by population interventions. *Lancet.* 1988; ii: 839.

Registrar General's Mortality (Cause) Statistics 1961 to 1995.

Fehily A M, *et al.* Diet and incident ischaemic heart disease: the Caerphilly Study. *Br J Nutr* 1993; 69: 303.

Shibata H, Nagai H, Haga H, Yasumura S, Suzuki T, Suyama Y. Nutrition for the Japanese elderly. *Nutr. Health.* 1992; 8(2-3): 165-75.

McMichael J M. Fats and atheroma: an inquest. *Br Med J.* 1979; 279: 890.

Bachorik P S, Cloey T A, Finney C A, Lowry D R, Becker D M. Lipoprotein-cholesterol analysis during screening: accuracy and reliability. *Ann Int Med.* 1991; 114: 741.

Myers G L, *et al.* College of American Pathologists – Centres for Disease Control collaborative study for evaluating reference materials for total serum cholesterol measurement. *Arch Pathol Lab Med.* 1990; 114: 1199-1205.

Sharp I, Rayner M. Cholesterol testing with desk-top machines. *Lancet.* 1990; i: 55.

Chapter 5: Is Exercise Necessary?

Prentice A M, Jebb S A. Obesity in Britain: gluttony or sloth? *Br Med J.* 1995; 311: 437-9

Björntorp P, *et al.* Physical training in human hyperplasic obesity. IV: Effects on hormonal status. *Metab.* 1977; 26: 319.

Krotkiewski M, *et al.* Effects of long-term physical training on body fat, metabolism, and blood pressure in obesity. *Metab.* 1979; 28: 650.

Yale J-F, Leiter L A, Marliss E B. Metabolic responses to intense exercise in lean and obese subjects. *J Clin Endocrin Metab.* 1989; 68: 438-45.

Oomura Y, Tarui S, Inoue S, Shimazu T, eds. *Progress in Obesity Research.* 1990, p 563. John Libby, London, 1990.

Voorrips L E, et al. History of body weight and physical activity of elderly women differing in current physical activity. *Int J Obes.* 1992; 16: 199.

Pacy P J, *et al.* The energy cost of aerobic exercise in fed and fasted normal subjects. *Am J Clin Nutr.* 1985; 42: 764.

Rothwell N J, Stock N J. Regulation of energy balance. *Ann Rev Nutr.* 1981; 1: 235.

Reid R L, van Vugt D A. Weight-related changes in reproductive function. *Fertil Steril.* 1987; 48(6): 905.

Cumming D C, *et al.* Exercise and reproductive function in women. *Prog Clin Biol Res.* 1983; 117: 113.

— Defects in pulsatile release in normally menstruating runners. *J Clin Endocrin Metab.* 1985; 60(4): 810.

Schwartz B, *et al.* Exercise associated amenorrhea: a distinct entity? *Am J Obstet Gynecol.* 1981; 141: 662.

Editorial. Reduced testosterone and prolactin in male distance runners. *JAMA.* 1984; 252: 514.

Chalmer J, *et al.* Anorexia nervosa presenting as morbid exercising. *Lancet.* 1985; i: 286.

Coplan N L, Gleim G W, Nicholas J A. Exercise and sudden cardiac death. *Am Heart J.* 1988; 115(1) pt.1: 207.

Fonda J. *Jane Fonda's Workout Book.* Penguin, London. 1984.

Morris J N, *et al.* Vigorous exercise in leisure time and the incidence of coronary heart disease. *Lancet.* 1973; i: 333.

Wagner W. Exercise-induced Allergic Syndromes on the Increase. *Cleveland Clin J Med.* 1989; 56: 665.

Selye H. *The Stress of Life.* McGraw-Hill. New York. 1956.

— *Annual Report on Stress. Montreal.* Acta Inc. 1951; Selye H, Horava A. 1952, 1953; Selye H, Heuser G, 1954; M D Public, New York. 1955-56.

Sawrey W L, Weisz J D. An experimental method of producing gastric ulcers. *J Comp Physio Psychol.* 1956; 49: 269.

Solomon G F. *Psychophysiological aspects of rheumatoid arthritis and auto-immune disease.* In O W Hill, ed. *Modern Trends in Psychosomatic Medicine* – 2. Butterworths, London. 1970.

Ketelhut R, Losem C J, Messerli F H. Is a decrease in arterial pressure during long-term exercise caused by a fall in cardiac pump function? *Am Heart J.* 1994; 127(3): 567-71.

Chapter 6: Are You Really Overweight?

Arner P. Not all fat is alike. *Lancet.* 1998; 351: 1301.

Van Itallie T B. The liquid protein mayhem. *JAMA.* 1978; 240: 140.

Wadden T A, *et al.* The Cambridge Diet: more mayhem? *JAMA.* 1983; 250: 2283.

Sours H E, *et al.* Sudden death associated with very low calorie weight reduction regimes. *Am J Clin Nutr.* 1981; 34: 453.

Jebb S A, Goldberg G R. Efficacy of very low-energy diets and meal replacements in the treatment of obesity. *J Human Nutr Diet.* 1998; 11: 219.

Editorial. In praise of embonpoint. *Lancet.* 1987; ii: 491.

Han T S, *et al.* Quality of life in relation to overweight and body fat distribution. *Am J Public Hlth.* 1998; 88: 1814.

Rosenbaum M, Leibel R L, Hirsch J. Medical progress: obesity. *N Engl J Med.* 1997; 337: 396-407.

Muoio D M, *et al.* Effect of dietary fat on metabolic adjustments to maximal VO-2 and endurance in runners. *Med Sci Sports Exercise.* 1994; 26 (1): 81-88.

Chapter 8: Breakfast: The Most Important Meal of the Day

Heaton K W. Breakfast – do we need it? Report of a meeting of the Forum on Food and Health, 16 June 1989. *J R Soc Med.* 1989; 82: 770.

Thorn G W, Quinby J T, Clinton M Jr. A comparison of the metabolic effects of isocaloric meals of varying compositions with special reference to the prevention of postprandial hypoglycemic symptoms. *Ann Int Med.* 1943; XVIII: 913.

Orent-Keiles E, Hallman L F. *The Breakfast Meal in Relation to Blood Sugar Values.* US Department of Agriculture Circular No 827 (1949).

Lloyd H M, Rogers P J, Hedderley D I, Walker A F. Acute effects on mood and cognitive performance of breakfasts differing in fat and carbohydrate content. *Appetite.* 1996; 27: 151.

Pollitt E. Does breakfast make a difference in school? *J Am Diet Assoc.* 1995; 95: 1134.

Index

Recipe Index

Recipe Index (contd)